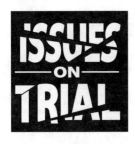

Disability Rights

Other Books in the Issues on Trial Series:

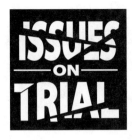

Disability Rights

Uma Kukathas, Book Editor

GREENHAVEN PRESS
A part of Gale, Cengage Learning

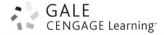

Detroit • New York • San Francisco • New Haven, Conn • Waterville, Maine • London

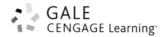
GALE
CENGAGE Learning™

Christine Nasso, *Publisher*
Elizabeth Des Chenes, *Managing Editor*

© 2010 Greenhaven Press, a part of Gale, Cengage Learning

For more information, contact:
Greenhaven Press
27500 Drake Rd.
Farmington Hills, MI 48331-3535
Or you can visit our Internet site at gale.cengage.com.

For product information and technology assistance, contact us at

Gale Customer Support, 1-800-877-4253
For permission to use material from this text or product, submit all requests online at www.cengage.com/permissions

Further permissions questions can be emailed to permissionrequest@cengage.com

Articles in Greenhaven Press anthologies are often edited for length to meet page requirements. In addition, original titles of these works are changed to clearly present the main thesis and to explicitly indicate the author's opinion. Every effort is made to ensure that Greenhaven Press accurately reflects the original intent of the authors. Every effort has been made to trace the owners of copyrighted material.

Cover photograph reproduced by permission of David McNew/Newsmakers/Getty Images.

LIBRARY OF CONGRESS CATALOGING-IN-PUBLICATION DATA

Disability rights / Uma Kukathas, book editor.
    p. cm. -- (Issues on trial)
Includes bibliographical references and index.
ISBN-13: 978-0-7377-4488-0 (hardcover)
1. People with disabilities--Legal status, laws, etc.--United States. 2. People with mental disabilities--Civil rights--United States. 3. Discrimination against people with disabilities--Law and legislation--United States. 4. Involuntary sterilization--United States. 5. Children with disabilities--Education--Law and legislation--United States. 6. Vocational rehabilitation--Law and legislation--United States. 7. People with disabilities--Services for--United States. I. Kukathas, Uma.
    KF480.D575 2009
    342.7308'7--dc22

                                                    2009019787

Printed in the United States of America
1 2 3 4 5 6 7 13 12 11 10 09

Contents

Chapter 2: Defining Free and Appropriate Education for Children of All Abilities

Chapter 3: Affirming the Rights of Disabled People to Participate in Community Life

Foreword

The U.S. courts have long served as a battleground for the most highly charged and contentious issues of the time. Divisive matters are often brought into the legal system by activists who feel strongly for their cause and demand an official resolution. Indeed, subjects that give rise to intense emotions or involve closely held religious or moral beliefs lay at the heart of the most polemical court rulings in history. One such case was *Brown v. Board of Education* (1954), which ended racial segregation in schools. Prior to *Brown*, the courts had held that blacks could be forced to use separate facilities as long as these facilities were equal to that of whites.

For years many groups had opposed segregation based on religious, moral, and legal grounds. Educators produced heartfelt testimony that segregated schooling greatly disadvantaged black children. They noted that in comparison to whites, blacks received a substandard education in deplorable conditions. Religious leaders such as Martin Luther King Jr. preached that the harsh treatment of blacks was immoral and unjust. Many involved in civil rights law, such as Thurgood Marshall, called for equal protection of all people under the law, as their study of the Constitution had indicated that segregation was illegal and un-American. Whatever their motivation for ending the practice, and despite the threats they received from segregationists, these ardent activists remained unwavering in their cause.

Those fighting against the integration of schools were mainly white southerners who did not believe that whites and blacks should intermingle. Blacks were subordinate to whites, they maintained, and society had to resist any attempt to break down strict color lines. Some white southerners charged that segregated schooling was *not* hindering blacks' education. For example, Virginia attorney general J. Lindsay Almond asserted, "With the help and the sympathy and the love and re-spect of the white people of the South, the colored man has risen under that educational process to a place of eminence and respect throughout the nation. It has served him well." So when the Supreme Court ruled against the segregationists in *Brown*, the South responded with vociferous cries of protest. Even government leaders criticized the decision. The governor of Arkansas, Orval Faubus, stated that he would not "be a party to any attempt to force acceptance of change to which the people are so overwhelmingly opposed." Indeed, resistance to integration was so great that when black students arrived at the formerly all-white Central High School in Arkansas, fed-eral troops had to be dispatched to quell a threatening mob of protesters.

Nevertheless, the *Brown* decision was enforced and the South integrated its schools. In this instance, the Court, while not settling the issue to everyone's satisfaction, functioned as an instrument of progress by forcing a major social change. Historian David Halberstam observes that the *Brown* ruling "deprived segregationist practices of their moral legitimacy. . . . It was therefore perhaps the single most important moment of the decade, the moment that separated the old order from the new and helped create the tumultuous era just arriving." Considered one of the most important victories for civil rights, *Brown* paved the way for challenges to racial segregation in many areas, including on public buses and in restaurants.

In examining *Brown*, it becomes apparent that the courts play an influential role—and face an arduous challenge—in shaping the debate over emotionally charged social issues. Judges must balance competing interests, keeping in mind the high stakes and intense emotions on both sides. As exempli-fied by *Brown*, judicial decisions often upset the status quo and initiate significant changes in society. Greenhaven Press's Issues on Trial series captures the controversy surrounding in-fluential court rulings and explores the social ramifications of such decisions from varying perspectives. Each anthology highlights one social issue—such as the death penalty, students' rights, or wartime civil liberties. Each volume then focuses on key historical and contemporary court cases that helped mold the issue as we know it today. The books include a compendium of primary sources—court rulings, dissents, and immediate reactions to the rulings—as well as secondary sources from experts in the field, people involved in the cases, legal analysts, and other commentators opining on the implications and legacy of the chosen cases. An annotated table of contents, an in-depth introduction, and prefaces that overview each case all provide context as readers delve into the topic at hand. To help students fully probe the subject, each volume contains book and periodical bibliographies, a comprehensive index, and a list of organizations to contact. With these features, the Issues on Trial series offers a well-rounded perspective on the courts' role in framing society's thorniest, most impassioned debates.

Introduction

In American society, individuals with disabilities have widely been viewed as deserving of charity and benevolence. As early as the nineteenth century, organizations providing for the care of people with disabilities were established in the United States. In 1817 the American School for the Deaf was founded in Hartford, Connecticut. Fifteen years later, in 1832, the Perkins School for the Blind in Boston admitted its first two students. In 1864 the Columbia Institution for the Deaf and Dumb and Blind became the first college in the world expressly established for people with disabilities. President Abraham Lincoln supported the cause by providing assistance for amputees returning home by the thousands from the Civil War.

To say that individuals with disabilities have been deemed worthy of charity, however, is not to say they have been deemed worthy of respect or equal opportunity and treatment as citizens. Indeed, too often they were not deemed worthy of citizenship at all. In 1883 Sir Francis Galton in England coined the term "eugenics" to describe his strategy for "improving the stock" of humanity. The eugenics movement, taken up in America, and among whose adherents included President Theodore Roosevelt, led to the passage in the United States of laws to prevent people with disabilities from moving to the country, marrying, or from having children. The side-by-side existence of noble acts of kindness and good will with shameful practices of discrimination, exclusion, and even oppression characterizes the history of disability in the United States.

To illustrate, in 1927, the same year that President Franklin Roosevelt established the Warm Springs Foundation for polio survivors, the U.S. Supreme Court ruled on *Buck v. Bell*. In *Buck*, the Court was asked to judge the constitutionality of a Virginia law permitting the forced sterilization of "feeble-minded" individuals. Those who favored the practice argued that selective breeding could greatly improve the health and overall quality of society by reducing the prevalence of feeble-mindedness, criminality, and other socially undesirable characteristics, which were believed to be inherited. The Supreme Court agreed, allowing the sterilization of Carrie Buck, a seventeen-year-old woman who had been confined to a state home, along with her mother and daughter, both of whom were also judged mentally and morally diminished. Although Buck's lawyer had argued that her full bodily integrity was protected by the Fourteenth Amendment, she lost her case. Chief Justice Oliver Wendell Holmes Jr., known as a champion of liberties, wrote the opinion in which he declared that society was better off without "imbeciles" and thus ought to "prevent their propagation by medical means." Such sterilization to prevent the birth of the "unfit" was compared to the use of vaccines to prevent smallpox; both could be forced on non-consenting citizens for the sake of the public's health and well-being.

Though never repealed, this law allowing states to interfere with fundamental freedoms of people with disabilities lacks force today. Although the eugenics movement was powerful in the 1920s and 1930s, advances in genetic science and revelations of Nazi atrocities discredited it and cemented in American minds the value of respect for individual autonomy. After the Second World War, returning veterans and the polio epidemic also brought attention to the needs of people with disabilities. These events underscored the need to define and protect the fundamental rights of persons with disabilities and thus planted seeds for changes that would bloom in the following decades.

The disability rights movement gained ground after the broader civil rights advances of the 1960s. Beginning with the Rehabilitation Act of 1973 it became an increasingly powerful force as its agendas gained recognition in legislation. The passage of the Rehabilitation Act of 1973 is often seen as the greatest achievement of the disability rights movement in confronting discrimination against people with disabilities. The act prohibits programs receiving federal funds from discriminating against "otherwise qualified handicapped" individuals. Its passage led, in turn, to a number of important regulations aimed at implementing the directive.

Before 1975 children with disabilities were largely excluded from public education. In 1972 the U.S. District Court for the District of Columbia, in *Mills v. Board of Education,* ruled that the District of Columbia could exclude children with disabilities from public schools. Other similar right-to-education decisions were used in public hearings leading to the passage of the Education for All Handicapped Children Act (EAHCA) of 1975. The EAHCA required that all public schools accepting federal funds provide equal access to "free appropriate public education" for children with physical and mental disabilities. When called on to interpret this requirement, the Supreme Court, in *Hendrick Hudson School District v. Rowley,* ruled that an "appropriate" education was neither a maximum education that would allow students with disabilities to reach their full potential nor an education that allowed these students to gain the same level of benefits available to other students. Instead, Justice William Rehnquist argued, schools must provide only a "basic floor of opportunity," one that provided "some benefit" to all students. Though not an entirely sufficient indicator of benefit, a student's passing from grade to grade was regarded as good evidence of adequate educational benefit. (This guideline, some observers report, creates an incentive for schools in need of federal funds to pass students regardless of their progress.) Though *Rowley* still stands as the legal precedent, in 1990 Congress reauthorized the EAHCA as the Individuals with Disabilities Education Act (IDEA), which imposes higher standards for what constitutes a free appropriate public education.

The treatment of persons with mental illness in the United States has changed dramatically since the nineteenth century. Some of the first health care facilities for the mentally ill were built and run by private associations. Many were progressive. At Vermont's Brattleboro Retreat, built in 1834, for example, patients produced their own newspaper, ran their own companies, and could join sports leagues, work the farm, or sing in a choir. State-run hospitals and institutions, however, did not provide their residents with such opportunities. The shortcomings of these facilities were highlighted in the 1940s, when many cases of patient abuse were documented by conscientious objectors assigned to psychiatric hospitals during World War II. In 1946 they founded the National Mental Health Foundation, whose mission was to expose the abusive conditions at those facilities. First Lady Eleanor Roosevelt came to be a strong supporter of the cause.

This is not to say that all mental health care institutions were terrible. Some played, and still play, an important, and even empowering, role in helping people with disabilities. Still, even facilities that provide competent and humane patient care can have the negative side-effect of unnecessarily segregating persons with disabilities from the rest of society. The Americans with Disabilities Act (ADA) of 1990 reflects this concern by requiring public agencies to undertake "reasonable modifications" to provide their services "in the most integrated setting appropriate to the needs of qualified individuals with disabilities." The constitutionality of this law was challenged, however. In *Olmstead v. L.C.* (1999), two women who had been voluntarily committed to a state-run hospital in Atlanta, Georgia, asked permission to leave after their conditions had improved. Although their doctors approved their request, the state would not release them. The Atlanta Legal Aid Society filed suit on their behalf, arguing that the ADA requires that the women be cared for in the most integrated setting possible. Justice Ruth Bader Ginsburg agreed with the plaintiffs. She argued that unnecessary institutionalization becomes a form of discrimination when it limits everyday freedoms or perpetuates the false perception that a patient is "incapable or unworthy of participating in community life." This ruling was seen by many as important for raising awareness of ways in which society unnecessarily excludes the mentally handicapped.

The basic architecture of public buildings and of infrastructure in general have had an exclusionary effect on people with disabilities. Consequently, in addition to its "integration mandate," the ADA also requires that local, state, and federal governments make reasonable modifications to ensure that their programs and services are accessible to persons with disabilities. This requirement of the ADA was challenged after two paraplegics filed suit against the state of Tennessee because the state's court buildings were not wheelchair accessible (*Tennessee v. Lane*, 2004). Again, the Court supported the ADA. Justice John Paul Stevens, writing for the majority, ruled that public agencies need to make sure their buildings and services can actually be used by persons with disabilities. Interestingly, the concerns raised in this case connect with the broad issues raised in *Buck v. Bell*. How much can be reasonably asked of one citizen, or group, in order to improve or establish the enjoyment of a right by another individual or group? Here the courts have been careful to carefully weigh out the benefits and burdens one issue at a time, rather than to make sweeping pronouncements. In *Tennessee v. Lane*, Stevens argued that reasonable accommodations are warranted in light of a long history of "pervasive unequal treatment in the administration of state services and programs."

The history of the disability rights movement reflects society's changing perceptions and interpretations of what it means to be disabled and what it means to guarantee persons with disabilities their full complement of constitutional rights. New technologies and changing social patterns are among the factors that give rise to the need to revise society's understanding, but many of the fundamental issues raised in earlier eras continue to be debated to this day. One thing is certain, however: the proper treatment of persons with disabilities is no longer just a question of defining society's charitable obligations but an issue of all its members' legal and moral rights.

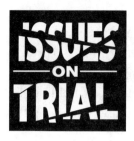

CHAPTER 1

Restricting the Rights of "Manifestly Unfit" Peoples to Reproduce

Case Overview

Buck v. Bell (1927)

The cultural roots of *Buck v. Bell* are found in the American eugenics movement of the early twentieth century. Eugenics proponents sought to improve society by encouraging the strong to breed while making sure the weak could not. They believed that traits like laziness, thievery, and sexual promiscuity were passed down from parent to child. Thousands of case studies were compiled to support these views. Organizations such as the American Eugenics Society presented eugenics exhibits at state fairs, and worked tirelessly to promote their cause. Their most famous supporter was president Theodore Roosevelt.

In 1924 the state of Virginia passed the Eugenical Sterilization Act. The act legalized compulsory sterilizations to rid Virginia of "defective persons." As soon as the law was passed, Albert Priddy, superintendent for the Virginia Colony for the Epileptic and Feebleminded, offered the law's first challenge. Priddy had been performing sterilizations on his wards for years. He believed that the most humane and cost-effective way to improve society was not to confine undesirables but to prevent them from reproducing. He hoped his legal challenge would be easily defeated and would thus strengthen the act's legality.

Carrie Buck had been committed to the asylum by her foster parents after she had given birth to an illegitimate child. (The fact that she had been raped by a relative of her foster parents was never revealed at trial.) Carrie's mother, Emma, had been committed years earlier. The case was first brought before the Circuit Court of Amherst County. Dozens of witnesses were called forward to testify to Carrie's feeblemindedness, including a former teacher who reported that Carrie had passed flirtatious notes to schoolboys. This was seen as evidence of her inherited promiscuity. The Amherst Circuit Court affirmed the validity of the sterilization law.

By 1927 the case had made its way to the U.S. Supreme Court. (By this time, Priddy had died, and his name was replaced on the case by that of the new superintendent, J.H. Bell.) By a vote of eight- to- one, the Court accepted the lower court's findings that Carrie Buck was "the probable parent of socially inadequate offspring . . . [and] that she may be sterilized without detriment to her general health and that her welfare and that of society will be promoted by her sterilization." In his opinion, Chief Justice Oliver Wendell Holmes Jr. relied on an earlier case, *Jacobson v. Massachusetts* (1905), which upheld a Massachusetts law requiring schoolchildren to be vaccinated against smallpox. In both cases, public welfare triumphed over individual liberties.

Immediately after the 1927 decision, there was a dramatic increase in the number of forced sterilizations nationwide. By the early 1930s thirty states had also passed eugenics laws. The eugenic-sterilization movement fared poorly in subsequent decades, however. In *Skinner v. Oklahoma* (1942), the Court accepted an equal protection challenge to Oklahoma's statute that provided for the sterilization of some habitual criminals. (Habitual white-collar criminals were exempted.) A few years later the horrors of the Nazi eugenics programs were revealed. This effectively squelched American social interest in anything resembling eugenics. Most states abandoned their sterilization laws in the 1950s. Virginia repealed its law in 1974. In 2002 the Virginia General Assembly passed a resolution honoring the memory of Carrie Buck. It states: "Legal and historical scholarship analyzing the *Buck* decision has condemned it as an embodiment of bigotry against the disabled and an example of using faulty science in support of public policy." The Supreme Court, however, has lacked the legal opportunity to overturn *Buck v. Bell*.

> *"It is better for all the world if, instead of waiting to execute degenerate offspring for crime or to let them starve for their imbecility, society can prevent those who are manifestly unfit from continuing their kind."*

Majority Opinion: The Mentally Unfit Can Be Forcibly Sterilized

Oliver Wendell Holmes Jr.

Oliver Wendell Holmes Jr., son of the poet Oliver Wendell Holmes, was appointed to the Supreme Court in 1902 by Theodore Roosevelt. He was much admired by progressives during his tenure because of his judicial restraint, championing of liberties, and view that free speech should not be curtailed by the government except in extreme cases. Holmes is probably the most frequently quoted Supreme Court justice, known for his aphorisms and pithy opinions. His opinion in Buck v. Bell *is characteristically brief at just over a thousand words. In the case, a young woman, Carrie Buck, who had been involuntarily institutionalized, claimed that the Virginia facility that sought to forcibly sterilize her was violating her constitutional rights. Buck had been deemed "feeble minded," along with her mother and seven-month-old infant daughter, and the colony where she was held argued that Buck would cease to be a charge on society if she could no longer reproduce. Her lawyer, Irving Whitehead, claimed that his client's "full bodily integrity" was protected by the Fourteenth Amendment and argued that if there were no*

Oliver Wendell Holmes Jr., majority opinion, *Buck v. Bell*, U.S. Supreme Court, 1927.

limits on the power of the state to rid itself of "undesirable" citizens, the worst type of tyranny would ensue. Holmes, writing for an eight-to-one majority, upheld as constitutional the Virginia statute that allowed compulsory sterilization of "mental defectives," women and men considered "unfit [to] continue their kind." Writing for the court, Holmes explains that sterilization is in the best interests of patients and society since heredity plays an important role in insanity and "imbecility." The justice evokes the notion that the nation's best give their lives for their countries in war, and thus those "incompetents" who sap the strength of the state should make a "lesser sacrifice" and not produce children who are bound to be criminals and imbeciles and thus burden the state. The single dissenting justice, Pierce Butler, did not write an opinion.

This is a writ of error to review a judgment of the Supreme Court of Appeals of the State of Virginia affirming a judgment of the Circuit Court of Amherst County by which the defendant in error, the superintendent of the State Colony for Epileptics and Feeble Minded, was ordered to perform the operation of salpingectomy [cutting and tying off the fallopian tubes] upon Carrie Buck, the plaintiff in error, for the purpose of making her sterile. The case comes here upon the contention that the statute authorizing the judgment is void under the *Fourteenth Amendment* as denying to the plaintiff in error due process of law and the equal protection of the laws.

Carrie Buck is a feeble minded white woman who was committed to the State Colony above mentioned in due form. She is the daughter of a feeble minded mother in the same institution, and the mother of an illegitimate feeble minded child. She was eighteen years old at the time of the trial of her case in the Circuit Court, in the latter part of 1924. An Act of Virginia, approved March 20, 1924, recites that the health of the patient and the welfare of society may be promoted in certain cases by the sterilization of mental defectives, under careful safeguard, &c. [etc.]; that the sterilization may be effected in males by vasectomy and in females by salpingectomy, without serious pain or substantial danger to life; that the Commonwealth is supporting in various institutions many defective persons who, if now discharged, would become a menace, but, if incapable of procreating, might be discharged with safety and become self-supporting with benefit to themselves and to society, and that experience has shown that heredity plays an important part in the transmission of insanity, imbecility, &c. The statute then enacts that, whenever the superintendent of certain institutions, including the above-named State Colony, shall be of opinion that it is for the best interests of the patients and of society that an inmate under his care should be sexually sterilized, he may have the operation performed upon any patient afflicted with hereditary forms of insanity, imbecility, &c., on complying with the very careful provisions by which the act protects the patients from possible abuse.

Rights of the Patient Considered

The superintendent first presents a petition to the special board of directors of his hospital or colony, stating the facts and the grounds for his opinion, verified by affidavit. Notice of the petition and of the time and place of the hearing in the institution is to be served upon the inmate, and also upon his guardian, and if there is no guardian, the superintendent is to apply to the Circuit Court of the County to appoint one. If the inmate is a minor, notice also is to be given to his parents, if any, with a copy of the petition. The board is to see to it that the inmate may attend the hearings if desired by him or his guardian. The evidence is all to be reduced to writing, and, after the board has made its order for or against the operation, the superintendent, or the inmate, or his guardian, may appeal to the Circuit Court of the County. The Circuit Court may consider the record of the board and the evidence before it and such other admissible evidence as may be offered, and may affirm, revise, or reverse the order of the board and enter such order as it deems just. Finally any party may apply to the Supreme Court of Appeals, which, if it grants the appeal, is to hear the case upon the record of the trial in the Circuit Court, and may enter such order as it thinks the Circuit Court should have entered. There can be no doubt that, so far as procedure is concerned, the rights of the patient are most carefully considered, and, as every step in this case was taken in scrupulous compliance with the statute and after months of observation, there is no doubt that, in that respect, the plaintiff in error has had due process of law.

Public Welfare

The attack is not upon the procedure, but upon the substantive law. It seems to be contended that in no circumstances could such an order be justified. It certainly is contended that the order cannot be justified upon the existing grounds. The judgment finds the facts that have been recited, and that Carrie Buck

> is the probable potential parent of socially inadequate offspring, likewise afflicted, that she may be sexually sterilized without detriment to her general health, and that her welfare and that of society will be promoted by her sterilization,

and thereupon makes the order. In view of the general declarations of the legislature and the specific findings of the Court, obviously we cannot say as matter of law that the grounds do not exist, and, if they exist, they justify the result. We have seen more than once that the public welfare may call upon the best citizens for their lives. It would be strange if it could not call upon those who already sap the strength of the State for these lesser sacrifices, often not felt to be such by those concerned, in order to prevent our being swamped with incompetence. It is better for all the world if, instead of waiting to execute degenerate offspring for crime or to let them starve for their imbecility, society can prevent those who are manifestly unfit from continuing their kind. The principle that sustains compulsory vaccination is broad enough to cover cutting the Fallopian tubes. Three generations of imbeciles are enough.

But, it is said, however it might be if this reasoning were applied generally, it fails when it is confined to the small number who are in the institutions named and is not applied to the multitudes outside. It is the usual last resort of constitutional arguments to point out shortcomings of this sort. But the answer is that the law does all that is needed when it does all that it can, indicates a policy, applies it to all within the lines, and seeks to bring within the lines all similarly situated so far and so fast as its means allow. Of course, so far as the operations enable those who otherwise must be kept confined to be returned to the world, and thus open the asylum to others, the equality aimed at will be more nearly reached.

Judgment affirmed.

"If one accepts as a major premise that
the state can demand of its citizens the
supreme sacrifice, it is a simple matter
for tyrants and logicians alike to reach
the conclusion reached here by Holmes."

Buck v. Bell Set a
Dangerous Precedent

Walter Berns

*Walter Berns is John M. Olin University Professor Emeritus at
Georgetown University and a resident scholar at the American
Enterprise Institute. His analysis of* Buck v. Bell, *a case in which
the Supreme Court found it constitutional to forcibly sterilize
people who were considered "unfit" to reproduce, was written in
1953, when forced sterilizations were still taking place around
the country. In his discussion he first takes issue with the idea
that the decision constituted a return to the "true" meaning of
the Constitution's Due Process Clause simply because the Virginia act of 1924 on which the sterilization law was based safe-
guarded procedural rights. He then goes on to provide the background to the forced sterilization movement in the United States
against which the* Buck v. Bell *trial took place. He shows how
influential the movement was on the public, the legislature, and
ultimately the Supreme Court. Berns also compares the American eugenicist ideas with the Nazi policies of planned race extinction, showing how the two were not very different in terms of
their science and philosophical underpinnings.*

Walter Berns, "*Buck v. Bell*: Due Process of Law?" *The Western Political Quarterly*, vol. 6,
no. 4, December 1953, pp. 762–74. Copyright © 1953. Reproduced by permission of
Sage Publications, Inc.

A quarter of a century has passed since Justice [Oliver Wendell] Holmes provided the eugenical sterilization movement with a constitutional blessing and an epigrammatic battle cry. His opinion for the Court in *Buck v. Bell* was regarded by eugenicists as the herald of a new day, and was joined in by all his brethren except Justice [Pierce] Butler. Whether the latter believed three generations of imbeciles were *not* enough, or that the number of generations was immaterial, we do not know, for while he did not withhold his judgment, he kept his reasons for dissenting to himself. The eugenicists, on the other hand, were anything but silent. Holmes, the subject of so much adulation, was hailed by them as the new Prometheus, and excerpts from his opinion continue to this day to add spice to their literature.

More than Procedures

Among political scientists concerned with constitutional law, the decision seems to have been implicitly accepted as a return to the "true" meaning of the due process clause. In his annual review of the Court's activities, Professor [R.E.] Cushman commented:

> The Virginia act of 1924, which was attacked, had carefully safeguarded procedural rights of those subject to the law so that no want of due process was made out on that score. The substance of the law itself is upheld as a reasonable social protection, entirely compatible with due process of law. Mr. Justice Holmes' trenchant statement of this warrants quotation.

He then proceeded to quote at length what is surely one of the most "totalitarian" statements in the history of the Court. The relevant part reads:

> We have seen more than once that the public welfare may call upon the best citizens for their lives. It would be strange if it could not call upon those who already sap the strength

of the State for these lesser sacrifices . . . in order to prevent our being swamped with incompetence.

If one accepts as a major premise that the state can demand of its citizens the supreme sacrifice, it is a simple matter for tyrants and logicians alike to reach the conclusion reached here by Holmes, that the state can then demand every lesser sacrifice. But American government, and all non-tyrannical government, is based on the recognition that there are greater evils than death. . . .

It is unfortunate that from a decision incorporating this view Justice Butler dissented without comment. The point should have been made, particularly for those who dissented so vigorously from the Field interpretation of it, that due process of law *does* require more than certain procedures, and that there are some things which decent government simply should not do. One of these is to perform compulsory surgical operations in order to satisfy the racial theories of a few benighted persons. To reduce the due process clause to a guarantee of prescribed procedures is to permit more than the public control of grain elevators, as libertarians since the *Gitlow* [*v. New York*] case would be the first to acknowledge. A restricted interpretation of the clause would have prevented the Court from interfering with Mayor [Frank] Hague's brand of tyranny in Jersey City [Hague was known for political favoritism and a form of social welfare known as bossism] and with those local school boards which have compelled children to salute the flag. If in the nineteenth century state legislatures were passing laws which won the favor of the liberal critics of the Court, they have, in the twentieth century, all too frequently passed laws which strike the same critics as gross violations of justice. The liberals' quarrel should be with injustice, not with the legal concept of substantive due process. Without the latter it would sometimes be impossible to prevent the former.

Tacit Acceptance

Prior to *Buck v. Bell*, the sterilization laws of seven states had been struck down by the courts, mostly for procedural reasons, but the Virginia statute under which Carrie Buck was to lose her ability to have children steered a prudent course around these reefs and arrived in Washington fairly glistening with safeguards for the individual: notice, hearing, counsel, and appeal by right to the courts. Such solicitude may have impressed Butler. Certainly it was not his habit to be overawed by Holmes, and if he had really believed that there was something inherently wrong in a law which compelled a person to be deprived of what can surely be numbered among the basic rights, he could have extrapolated something from her counsel's brief to support some kind of dissent. Certainly Holmes's argument that "The principle that sustains compulsory vaccination is broad enough to cover cutting the Fallopian tubes. . . ." should not have been permitted to escape at least examination. It is a broad principle indeed that sustains a needle's prick in the arm and an abdominal incision, if only in terms of the equipment used. It becomes something else again in terms of the results attained: no smallpox in the one case and no children in the other.

Perhaps the Court's position was not easy. The eugenicists had painted so lurid and so convincing a picture of an unsterilized America, with the Carrie Bucks and their offspring cluttering the scene like germs under the microscope in the Listerine advertisement, that even their opponents, however few in number at the time, were disquieted. Furthermore, no one, not even her counsel, challenged the eugenical account; no civil liberties organization sprang forward to defend Carrie, yet one would assume that children are as basic to the nation's needs as speech. Nor is it even necessary to elevate children to a "preferred position," or take an intransigent stand on natural rights, to disagree with this decision; a true pragmatist could have dissented just as well.

Holmes, however, was following his "ideal for the law" when he said, ". . . if they [the grounds for sterilization] exist they justify the result." But as [critic John B. Guest] has written, "Justice Holmes assumes the efficacy of sterilization, a judgment on which would be worthy of a minor prophet." It would be more accurate to say that the Court assumed that the legislature possessed this gift of prophecy, which was an unwarranted assumption in this case. It was impossible to discover how intensive the hearings before the legislative committee had been, but the record of the litigation shows that the state tribunal, the Virginia Supreme Court of Appeals, had probed no deeper into the substance of the eugenical argument than Holmes had; it merely accepted without question the evidence submitted by Bell, the superintendent of the state institution, and the testimony of his witnesses at the hearing of the special board. The court then said: "Carrie Buck, by the laws of heredity, is the probable potential parent of socially inadequate offspring likewise affected as she is."

To a considerable extent the court was able to escape the responsibility for examining these so-called "laws of heredity" because of the failure of Carrie Buck's counsel to force such an evaluation. Someone should have looked into the "probability of the potentiality of the inadequacy"; but at no time during the litigation, from the hearing before the special board to the brief he submitted to the Supreme Court of the United States, did Counsel [Irving] Whitehead offer any evidence or produce any witness to question the validity of the eugenical basis of the statute. Perhaps there was no evidence available to him at the time, for, while Bell produced scientists, physicians, nurses, and other people who had known Carrie Buck, not one witness came forward on Carrie's behalf. It may be that only on the basis of knowledge available later could he have cast doubt on the relevance of Mendel's peas to the problem of human heredity [Gregor Mendel, often referred to as the father of genetics, conducted a study using pea plants to examine the inheritance of traits], or attacked the deposition of Dr. H. H. Laughlin, one of the leaders of the sterilization movement, who pronounced Carrie feeble-minded without ever having seen her, or produced a witness to show that the "scientific evidence" was mere fabrication, or at most supposition; perhaps his ineffectual questions directed at subsidiary aspects of the case were the only ones available to him. It may be true that the case handed him was indeed a hopeless one.

Ridding the World of Carrie Bucks

It was certainly a good one for Bell. Carrie was doubtless feeble-minded. R. G. Shelton, her "next friend," was actually a guardian appointed, under the terms of the statute, by the Circuit Court of Amherst County, Virginia. Her counsel was hired by the State. She had no relatives except her feeble-minded mother who, as a ward of the State, was under supervision; no friends came forward to protest at any stage of the proceedings; there was no one who was vitally concerned in her welfare. Her illegitimate child was adjudged subnormal because it was not as "responsive" as the child of the woman who made the comparison! If ever the state of Virginia had a good case to push through the courts and a case likely to arouse the minimum of opposition, it was this case of friendless, feeble-minded Carrie Buck, who, in reply to this question put by Bell's counsel: "Do you care to say anything about having this operation performed on you?" said, "No, sir, I have not, it is up to my people"—whoever they were.

Bell's "people," on the other hand, were well known—at least in sterilization circles. Dr. Laughlin was out to rid the world of the Carrie Bucks, but also of the likes of Beethoven, Mozart, Milton, Poe, and Napoleon, to name only a few of the men who would have been sterilized under his "model law." Arthur H. Estabrook, who also testified for Bell, was the man who had "proved" the applicability of Mendel's pea-findings to human beings by his studies of the Jukes and Nam families.

A favorable decision from the Supreme Court was necessary for the fulfillment of their plans, and this case from Virginia was designed for that decision. As Dr. Laughlin put it, ". . . the Virginia statute is, in the main, one of the best laws thus far enacted in that it has avoided the principal eugenical and legal defects of previous statutes, and has incorporated into it the most effective eugenical features and the soundest legal principles of previous laws."

Although these litigants had technically adverse interests, this case, like so many others involving great constitutional issues, was probably a friendly one. Carrie Buck, to judge by the testimony in the hearing, had no quarrels with anyone; she simply was not very bright, which caused her to be a burden on the state and put her in a classification which Laughlin and Estabrook sought to eradicate from the American population. Holmes certified that such eradication was legal, but one is permitted to wonder if he would have been so cavalier in his certification if he had known the extent of the plans. Dr. Laughlin's plans called for the sterilization of 203,255 Americans annually by 1950, while estimating, according to a Mendelian thesis, that the number of "socially inadequate" persons, or persons capable of producing socially inadequate offspring, would total 11,891,700 in the same year! However the lines are drawn and the categories filled, this is a large section of the American people. . . .

The Sterilization Movement in America

What grievous conditions prevailed among the American people to justify the Laughlin program of hundreds of thousands of state-performed surgical operations annually? One woman, Mrs. E. H. Harriman, who apparently considered conditions grievous enough to warrant the gift of the Eugenics Record Office to doctors Laughlin and Davenport, once got up in a public meeting to shout, "What is the matter with the American people? 15,000,000 must be sterilized!" Not eleven, but fifteen million! But what were the symptoms, why must so many of us be sterilized? "The number of known mentally diseased persons is now three times as great in proportion to the total population, as it was in 1880." "America is breeding from the bottom." "Nature's plan is interfered with by human sympathy and modern charity." "Mentally deficient voters threaten democratic government." "Sterilization is a matter of national preservation." These are indeed grievous conditions, but what could be done about it? Just remove some "little bits of tubes." It is that simple. "... it is claimed that if sterilization laws could be enforced in the whole United States, less than four generations would eliminate nine-tenths of the feeble-mindedness, insanity and crime in the country." Even crime! O Brave New World! Can anyone protest its realization? . . .

It should be made clear that the men to be quoted in the following pages were not apostates [one who abandons a previous loyalty] but were the leaders of the sterilization movement in America; in fact, with no notable exceptions, they *were* the movement. They were the Cassandras [referring to the character in Greek mythology] whose dire prophecies frightened state legislators into voting for the bills they had composed and proposed. One of them had conducted the "research" which had led to the enthronement of three "royal families of feeble-mindedom," while others joined in the widespread lament for a soon-to-be-lost Anglo-Saxon world of their fathers. While joining the protest against the "new immigration," they were prepared to take harsher action if the quota system should prove inadequate. As for the Italians, Slavs, Poles, Jews, and Greeks already here . . . and what about the Negroes? Dr. Laughlin's model law was designed to deal with them all, as the Nazis, who translated it into German, proved.

Eugenics in America and Nazi Germany

Commenting on this model law, Dr. [Abraham] Myerson wrote: "Either the proponents of this legislation are naive beyond my simple powers of expression, or else—what?" It is now possible to answer this question in a way that might lead such organizations as the Federation of Women's Clubs and the American Association of University Women to reconsider their support of the sterilization cause.

To begin with, were Laughlin and Davenport thinking of mental defectives when they penned this editorial?

> Within its own territory each race must, by all humanity, be granted the right to promote its own race integrity. The right to strive for race integrity is like the pursuit of happiness. . . .
>
> When the European emigration waves after the World War were about to overwhelm America, President [Calvin] Coolidge said "America must remain American." Similarly, each race, whether the French at home, the Germans at home, the Jews in their new homeland . . . has an inherent right to set its own racial standards and to regulate immigration and human reproduction in such a manner as to breed toward the attainment of these standards.
>
> It is the business of eugenics, both as a pure and as an applied science in each country, to collaborate with its national leadership in establishing the racial and family-stock ideals for the particular country, and in striving for the attainment of the established ideals.

"Race integrity" and "regulate human reproduction!" The copies of the *Eugenical News* published under the editorship of Laughlin and Davenport are filled with phrases similar to these. Another editorial in the same year reads: "One may condemn the Nazi policy generally, but specifically it remained for Germany in 1933 to lead the great nations of the world in recognition of the biological foundations of national character." Nor do they content themselves with editorials. In 1934 they reprinted an entire speech by Dr. Frick, Reichsminister of the Interior, entitled: "German Population and Race Politics", and up until the time of the war the good news from Germany filled the pages of the magazine. The German law was reproduced, explained and, by a German here, interpreted:

> In the new Germany laws are made for the benefit of posterity, regardless of the approval or disapproval of present generations. . . .

> This [being swamped by degenerate stock] is the colossal danger Adolf Hitler wants to avert in Germany! A nation decays because its valuable germplasm disappears—that racial stock from which leaders emerge.

So that there can be no doubt where they stand, the editors, at the end of this article, write:

> Whether or not the critic agrees with current German ideas, real or reputed, the student of eugenics agrees that as practical statesmanship for effecting the announced ideals, Germany is the first of the great nations of the world to make direct use of eugenics. . . .

> To combat the rising tide of mental and physical defectives and to preserve the proper proportion of the Aryan elements in Germany the state is initiating many eugenic measures, including the sterilization law . . . and other measures *to eliminate the non-Aryan element from Germany.*

And in an unsigned book review in the same issue there appears this statement:

> It appears that under the dictatorship Germany is moving more rapidly toward race purification than any other nation. Such race purification may be accompanied by hardships to the individual, but society follows nature's method in regarding the progress of the race as more important than that of the individual.

For anyone still in doubt as to what these eugenicists had in mind for the American people when they spoke of human betterment, the bound volumes of the *Eugenical News* will provide enlightenment, and especially recommended is the article "Patriotism and Racial Standards" in the issue of July–August, 1936, written by C. M. Goethe, one of the current sponsors of the Human Betterment Association; but here, one more quotation will suffice:

> It is unfortunate the anti-Nazi propaganda with which all countries have been flooded has gone far to obscure the correct understanding and the great importance of the German racial policy. . . . No earnest eugenicist can fail to give approbation to such a national policy.

Who was the man who wrote this? He was the honorary president of the Eugenics Research Association. He ended the article with these words:

> The Germans as a nation recognize that these obligations in the common interest go somewhat further, and they are quite happy and content to observe such further obligations in the feeling that their personal liberties are not unduly curtailed. The future will incontestably prove which nations have been the wiser.

Whether it was the advent of the war, the attacks on the American Bund, or the end of the editorial reign of Laughlin and Davenport, the tone of the magazine had changed by 1939, and while the Nazi racial policy apparently was never repudiated, the magazine printed an article in 1943 which, after a recitation of some of Hitler's crimes, contained this statement: "These almost unbelievable facts bring to our hearts a rush of pity for those victims of sadism, brutality and planned race extinction."

The elimination of the non-Aryan element had turned out to be race extinction! But how in the name of the English language could it have turned out to be anything else? Where eugenical collaboration with national leadership had produced a "nordic" definition of *Volksgesundheit* [public health] in Germany, which in turn was eventually carried out in the gas chambers, who can be certain that these American eugenicists would not, finally, have been intrigued with this far more efficient method of sterilization? In Germany it was *ein Reich, ein Volk, ein Führer* [one nation, one people, one leader]; in America [Roswell Hill] Johnson and [eugenicist Paul] Popenoe were calling for an "Aristo-democracy." The difference may be one of terminology only.

Eugenic Sterilization Earned Its Justification on a Patent Falsehood

Stephen Jay Gould

Stephen Jay Gould was a noted American paleontologist, evolutionary biologist, and historian of science. In the following essay, he demonstrates that the premise of the case against Carrie Buck—that she was genetically defective because she was the daughter of an "imbecile" and gave birth to a "mentally retarded" child—was false. Gould shows that neither mother nor child was of anything but normal intelligence and that Carrie Buck was probably institutionalized not because of her diminished mental capacity but because she had a baby out of wedlock—the result of rape by a member of her foster family, which the family wanted to cover up. When the 1924 compulsory sterilization law in Virginia was passed, she was the first person selected for the procedure. Because she was the offspring of and the mother to supposed mental defectives, the state could thus argue the issue of inheritance of defective traits was central to the case. Gould provides evidence to show that Buck was certainly not mentally ill nor developmentally disabled, and that her daughter was likely of at least average intellectual ability. "Imbecility" in

Stephen Jay Gould, "Carrie Buck's Daughter," *Natural History*, vol. 93, July–August 2002, pp. 14–18. Copyright © the American Museum of Natural History 2002. Reproduced by permission.

the case was used as a cover-up for Buck's pregnancy, he maintains; the case was not about mental deficiency but about sexual morality.

The Lord really put it on the line in his preface to that prototype of all prescription, the Ten Commandments:

> for I, the Lord thy God, am a jealous God, visiting the iniquity of the fathers upon the children unto the third and fourth generation of them that hate me. (Exod. 20:5)

The terror of this statement lies in its patent unfairness—its promise to punish guiltless offspring for the misdeeds of their distant forebears.

A different form of guilt by genealogical association attempts to remove this stigma of injustice by denying a cherished premise of Western thought—human free will. If offspring are tainted not simply by the deeds of their parents but by a material form of evil transferred directly by biological inheritance, then "the iniquity of the fathers" becomes a signal or warning for probable misbehavior of their sons. Thus Plato, while denying that children should suffer directly for the crimes of their parents, nonetheless defended the banishment of a man whose father, grandfather, and great-grandfather had all been condemned to death.

It is, perhaps, merely coincidental that both Jehovah and Plato chose three generations as their criterion for establishing different forms of guilt by association. Yet we have a strong folk, or vernacular, tradition for viewing triple occurrences as minimal evidence of regularity. We are told that bad things come in threes. Two may be an accidental association; three is a pattern. Perhaps, then, we should not wonder that our own century's most famous pronouncement of blood guilt employed the same criterion—Oliver Wendell Holmes's defense of compulsory sterilization in Virginia (Supreme Court decision of 1927 in *Buck v. Bell*): "three generations of imbeciles are enough."

The Eugenics Movement

Restrictions upon immigration, with national quotas set to discriminate against those deemed mentally unfit by early versions of IQ testing, marked the greatest triumph of the American eugenics movement—the flawed hereditarian doctrine, so popular earlier in our century and by no means extinct today, that attempted to "improve" our human stock by preventing the propagation of those deemed biologically unfit and encouraging procreation among the supposedly worthy. But the movement to enact and enforce laws for compulsory "eugenic" sterilization had an impact and success scarcely less pronounced. If we could debar the shiftless and the stupid from our shores, we might also prevent the propagation of those similarly afflicted but already here.

The movement for compulsory sterilization began in earnest during the 1890s, abetted by two major factors—the rise of eugenics as an influential political movement and the perfection of safe and simple operations (vasectomy for men and salpingectomy, the cutting and tying of Fallopian tubes, for women) to replace castration and other obvious mutilation. Indiana passed the first sterilization act based on eugenic principles in 1907 (a few states had previously mandated castration as a punitive measure for certain sexual crimes, although such laws were rarely enforced and usually overturned by judicial review). Like so many others to follow, it provided for sterilization of afflicted people residing in the state's "care," either as inmates of mental hospitals and homes for the feebleminded or as inhabitants of prisons. Sterilization could be imposed upon those judged insane, idiotic, imbecilic, or moronic, and upon convicted rapists or criminals when recommended by a board of experts.

By the 1930s, more than thirty states had passed similar laws, often with an expanded list of so-called hereditary defects, including alcoholism and drug addiction in some states, and even blindness and deafness in others. It must be said that these laws were continually challenged and rarely enforced in most states; only California and Virginia applied them zealously. By January 1935, some 20,000 forced "eugenic" sterilizations had been performed in the United States, nearly half in California.

The Eugenics Record Office

No organization crusaded more vociferously and successfully for these laws than the Eugenics Record Office, the semiofficial arm and repository of data for the eugenics movement in America. Harry Laughlin, superintendent of the Eugenics Record Office, dedicated most of his career to a tireless campaign of writing and lobbying for eugenic sterilization. He hoped, thereby, to eliminate in two generations the genes of what he called the "submerged tenth"—"the most worthless one-tenth of our present population." He proposed a "model sterilization law" in 1922, designed

> to prevent the procreation of persons socially inadequate from defective inheritance, by authorizing and providing for eugenical sterilization of certain potential parents carrying degenerate hereditary qualities.

This model bill became the prototype for most laws passed in America, although few states cast their net as widely as Laughlin advised. (Laughlin's categories encompassed "blind, including those with seriously impaired vision; deaf, including those with seriously impaired hearing; and dependent, including orphans, ne'er-do-wells, the homeless, tramps, and paupers.") Laughlin's suggestions were better heeded in Nazi Germany, where his model act served as a basis for the infamous and stringently enforced Erbgesundheitsrecht [law of genetic health], leading by the eve of World War II to the sterilization of some 375,000 people, most for "congenital feeble-mindedness," but including nearly 4,000 for blindness and deafness.

Carrie Buck and Genetic Inheritance

The campaign for forced eugenic sterilization in America reached its climax and height of respectability in 1927, when the Supreme Court, by an 8-1 vote, upheld the Virginia sterilization bill in the case of *Buck v. Bell*. Oliver Wendell Holmes, then in his mid-eighties and the most celebrated jurist in America, wrote the majority opinion with his customary verve and power of style. It included the notorious paragraph, with its chilling tag line, cited ever since as the quintessential statement of eugenic principles. Remembering with pride his own distant experiences as an infantryman in the Civil War, Holmes wrote:

> We have seen more than once that the public welfare may call upon the best citizens for their lives. It would be strange if it could not call upon those who already sap the strength of the state for these lesser sacrifices. . . . It is better for all the world, if instead of waiting to execute degenerate offspring for crime, or to let them starve for their imbecility, society can prevent those who are manifestly unfit from continuing their kind. The principle that sustains compulsory vaccination is broad enough to cover cutting the Fallopian tubes. Three generations of imbeciles are enough.

Who, then, were the famous "three generations of imbeciles," and why should they still compel our interest?

When the state of Virginia passed its compulsory sterilization law in 1924, Carrie Buck, an eighteen-year-old white woman, was an involuntary resident at the State Colony for Epileptics and Feeble-Minded. As the first person selected for sterilization under the new act, Carrie Buck became the focus for a constitutional challenge launched, in part, by conservative Virginia Christians who held, according to eugenical "modernists," antiquated views about individual preferences and "benevolent" state power. (Simplistic political labels do not apply in this case, and rarely do in general. We usually regard eugenics as a conservative movement and its most vocal critics as members of the left. This alignment has generally held in our own decade. But eugenics, touted in its day as the latest in scientific modernism, attracted many liberals and numbered among its most vociferous critics groups often labeled as reactionary and antiscientific. If any political lesson emerges from these shifting allegiances, we might consider the true inalienability of certain human rights.) But why was Carrie Buck in the State Colony, and why was she selected? Oliver Wendell Holmes upheld her choice as judicious in the opening lines of his 1927 opinion:

> Carrie Buck is a feeble-minded white woman who was committed to the State Colony.... She is the daughter of a feeble-minded mother in the same institution, and the mother of an illegitimate feeble-minded child.

In short, inheritance stood as the crucial issue (indeed as the driving force behind all eugenics). For if measured mental deficiency arose from malnourishment, either of body or mind, and not from tainted genes, then how could sterilization be justified? If decent food, upbringing, medical care, and education might make a worthy citizen of Carrie Buck's daughter, how could the State of Virginia justify the severing of Carrie's Fallopian tubes against her will? (Some forms of mental deficiency are passed by inheritance in family line, but most are not—a scarcely surprising conclusion when we consider the thousand shocks that beset fragile humans during their lives, from difficulties in embryonic growth to traumas of birth, malnourishment, rejection, and poverty. In any case, no fair-minded person today would credit Laughlin's social criteria for the identification of hereditary deficiency—ne'er-do-wells, the homeless, tramps, and paupers—although we shall soon see that Carrie Buck was committed on these grounds.)

When Carrie Buck's case emerged as the crucial test of Virginia's law, the chief honchos of eugenics knew that the time had come to put up or shut up on the crucial issue of inheritance. Thus, the Eugenics Record Office sent Arthur H. Estabrook, their crack fieldworker, to Virginia for a "scientific" study of the case. Harry Laughlin himself provided a deposition, and his brief for inheritance was presented at the local trial that affirmed Virginia's law and later worked its way to the Supreme Court as *Buck v. Bell*.

The Cause of Feeblemindedness

Laughlin made two major points to the court. First, that Carrie Buck and her mother, Emma Buck, were feeble-minded by the Stanford-Binet test of IQ, then in its own infancy. Carrie scored a mental age of nine years, Emma of seven years and eleven months. (These figures ranked them technically as "imbeciles" by definitions of the day, hence Holmes's later choice of words. Imbeciles displayed a mental age of six to nine years; idiots performed worse, morons better, to round out the old nomenclature of mental deficiency.) Second, that most feeblemindedness is inherited, and Carrie Buck surely belonged with this majority. Laughlin reported:

> Generally feeble-mindedness is caused by the inheritance of degenerate qualities; but sometimes it might be caused by environmental factors which are not hereditary. In the case given, the evidence points strongly toward the feeble-mindedness and moral delinquency of Carrie Buck being due, primarily, to inheritance and not to environment.

Carrie Buck's daughter was then, and has always been, the pivotal figure of this painful case. As I stated before, we tend (often at our peril) to regard two as potential accident and three as an established pattern. The supposed imbecility of Emma and Carrie might have been coincidental, but the diagnosis of similar deficiency for Vivian Buck (made by a social worker, as we shall see, when Vivian was but six months old) tipped the balance in Laughlin's favor and led Holmes to declare the Buck lineage inherently corrupt by deficient heredity. Vivian sealed the pattern—three generations of imbeciles are enough. Besides, had Carrie not given illegitimate birth to Vivian, the issue (in both senses) would never have emerged.

Oliver Wendell Holmes viewed his work with pride. The man so renowned for his principle of judicial restraint, who had proclaimed that freedom must not be curtailed without "clear and present danger"—without the equivalent of falsely yelling "fire" in a crowded theater—wrote of his judgment in *Buck v. Bell*: "I felt that I was getting near the first principle of real reform."

Why Carrie Buck Was Really Committed

And so the case of *Buck v. Bell* remained for fifty years, a footnote to a moment of American history perhaps best forgotten. And then, in 1980, it reemerged to prick our collective conscience, when Dr. K. Ray Nelson, then director of the Lynchburg Hospital where Carrie Buck was sterilized, researched the records of his institution and discovered that more than 4,000 sterilizations had been performed, the last as late as 1972. He also found Carrie Buck, alive and well near Charlottesville, and her sister Doris, covertly sterilized under the same law (she was told that her operation was for appendicitis), and now, with fierce dignity, dejected and bitter because she had wanted a child more than anything else in her life and had finally, in her old age, learned why she had never conceived.

As scholars and reporters visited Carrie Buck and her sister, what a few experts had known all along became abundantly clear to everyone. Carrie Buck was a woman of obviously normal intelligence. For example, Paul A. Lombardo of the School of Law at the University of Virginia, and a leading scholar of the *Buck v. Bell* case, wrote in a letter to me:

> As for Carrie, when I met her she was reading newspapers daily and joining a more literate friend to assist at regular bouts with the crossword puzzles. She was not a sophisticated woman, and lacked social graces, but mental health

professionals who examined her in later life confirmed my impressions that she was neither mentally ill nor retarded.

On what evidence, then, was Carrie Buck consigned to the State Colony for Epileptics and Feeble-Minded on January 23, 1924? I have seen the text of her commitment hearing; it is, to say the least, cursory and contradictory. Beyond the simple and undocumented say-so of her foster parents, and her own brief appearance before a commission of two doctors and a justice of the peace, no evidence was presented. Even the crude and early Stanford-Binet test, so fatally flawed as a measure of innate worth but at least clothed with the aura of quantitative respectability, had not yet been applied.

When we understand why Carrie Buck was committed in January 1924, we can finally comprehend the hidden meaning of her case and its message for us today. The silent key, again and as always, is her daughter Vivian, born on March 28, 1924, and then but an evident bump on her belly. Carrie Buck was one of several illegitimate children borne by her mother, Emma. She grew up with foster parents, J.T. and Alice Dobbs, and continued to live with them, helping out with chores around the house. She was apparently raped by a relative of her foster parents, then blamed for her resultant pregnancy. Almost surely, she was (as they used to say) committed to hide her shame (and her rapist's identity), not because enlightened science had just discovered her true mental status. In short, she was sent away to have her baby. Her case never was about mental deficiency; it was always a matter of sexual morality and social deviance. The annals of her trial and hearing reek with the contempt of the well-off and well-bred for poor people of "loose morals." Who really cared whether Vivian was a baby of normal intelligence; she was the illegitimate child of an illegitimate woman. Two generations of bastards are enough. Harry Laughlin began his "family history" of the Bucks by writing: "These people belong to the shiftless, ignorant and worthless class of anti-social whites of the South."

"Imbecility" as a Cover-Up

We know little of Emma Buck and her life, but we have no more reason to suspect her than her daughter Carrie of true mental deficiency. Their deviance was social and sexual; the charge of imbecility was a cover-up, Mr. Justice Holmes notwithstanding.

We come then to the crux of the case, Carrie's daughter, Vivian. What evidence was ever adduced for her mental deficiency? This and only this: At the original trial in late 1924, when Vivian Buck was seven months old, a Miss Wilhelm, social worker for the Red Cross, appeared before the court. She began by stating honestly the true reason for Carrie Buck's commitment:

> Mr. Dobbs, who had charge of the girl, had taken her when a small child, had reported to Miss Duke [the temporary secretary of Public Welfare for Albemarle County] that the girl was pregnant and that he wanted to have her committed somewhere—to have her sent to some institution.

Miss Wilhelm then rendered her judgment of Vivian Buck by comparing her with the normal granddaughter of Mrs. Dobbs, born just three days earlier:

> It is difficult to judge probabilities of a child as young as that, but it seems to me not quite a normal baby. In its appearance—I should say that perhaps my knowledge of the mother may prejudice me in that regard, but I saw the child at the same time as Mrs. Dobbs' daughter's baby, which is only three days older than this one, and there is a very decided difference in the development of the babies. That was about two weeks ago. There is a look about it that is not quite normal, but just what it is, I can't tell.

This short testimony, and nothing else, formed all the evidence for the crucial third generation of imbeciles. Cross-examination revealed that neither Vivian nor the Dobbs grandchild could walk or talk, and that "Mrs. Dobbs' daughter's baby is a very responsive baby. When you play with it or try to attract its attention—it is a baby that you can play with. The other baby is not. It seems very apathetic and not responsive." Miss Wilhelm then urged Carrie Buck's sterilization: "I think," she said, "it would at least prevent the propagation of her kind." Several years later, Miss Wilhelm denied that she had ever examined Vivian or deemed the child feebleminded.

The Real Vivian Buck

Unfortunately, Vivian died at age eight of "enteric colitis" (as recorded on her death certificate), an ambiguous diagnosis that could mean many things but may well indicate that she fell victim to one of the preventable childhood diseases of poverty (a grim reminder of the real subject in *Buck v. Bell*). She is therefore mute as a witness in our reassessment of her famous case.

When *Buck v. Bell* resurfaced in 1980, it immediately struck me that Vivian's case was crucial and that evidence for the mental status of a child who died at age eight might best be found in report cards. I have therefore been trying to track down Vivian Buck's school records for the past four years and have finally succeeded. (They were supplied to me by Dr. Paul A. Lombardo, who also sent other documents, including Miss Wilhelm's testimony, and spent several hours answering my questions by mail and Lord knows how much time playing successful detective in re[gard to] Vivian's school records. I have never met Dr. Lombardo; he did all this work for kindness, collegiality, and love of the game of knowledge, not for expected reward or even requested acknowledgment. In a profession—academics—so often marked by pettiness and silly squabbling over meaningless priorities, this generosity must be recorded and celebrated as a sign of how things can and should be.)

Vivian Buck was adopted by the Dobbs family, who had raised (but later sent away) her mother, Carrie. As Vivian Alice Elaine Dobbs, she attended the Venable Public Elementary School of Charlottesville for four terms, from September 1930 until May 1932, a month before her death. She was a perfectly normal, quite average student, neither particularly outstanding nor much troubled. In those days before grade inflation, when C mean "good, 81–87" (as defined on her report card) rather than barely scraping by, Vivian Dobbs received A's and B's for deportment and C's for all academic subjects but mathematics (which was always difficult for her, and where she scored D) during her first term in Grade 1A, from September 1930 to January 1931. She improved during her second term in 1B, meriting an A in deportment, C in mathematics, and B in all other academic subjects; she was on the honor roll in April 1931. Promoted to 2A, she had trouble during the fall term of 1931, failing mathematics and spelling but receiving A in deportment, B in reading, and C in writing and English. She was "retained in 2A" for the next term—or "left back" as we used to say, and scarcely a sign of imbecility as I remember all my buddies who suffered a similar fate. In any case, she again did well in her final term, with B in deportment, reading, and spelling, and C in writing, English, and mathematics during her last month in school. This offspring of "lewd and immoral" women excelled in deportment and performed adequately, although not brilliantly, in her academic subjects.

In short, we can only agree with the conclusion that Dr. Lombardo has reached in his research on *Buck v. Bell*—there were no imbeciles, not a one, among the three generations of Bucks. I don't know that such correction of cruel but forgotten errors of history counts for much, but it is at least satisfying to learn that forced eugenic sterilization, a procedure of such dubious morality, earned its official justification (and won its most quoted line of rhetoric) on a patent falsehood.

Carrie Buck died [in 2001]. By a quirk of fate, and not by memory or design, she was buried just a few steps from her only daughter's grave. In the umpteenth and ultimate verse of a favorite old ballad, a rose and a brier—the sweet and the bitter—emerge from the tombs of Barbara Allen and her lover, twining about each other in the union of death. May Carrie and Vivian, victims in different ways and in the flower of youth, rest together in peace.

> *"Though society may be inclined to regard Holmes's detestable opinion in Buck v. Bell as a relic of a time past, eerie similarities exist in contemporary remarks of the well-respected."*

The Eugenicist Mindset Still Exists

Andrew J. Imparato and Anne C. Sommers

Andrew J. Imparato is president and chief executive of the American Association of People with Disabilities, and Anne C. Sommers is the legislative affairs specialist for the National Council on Disability. In the following essay they argue that while the science behind the decision in Buck v. Bell *has been clearly debunked, several renowned thinkers have made remarks about people with disabilities that echo those earlier views. In* Buck v. Bell *the plaintiff, Carrie Buck, claimed that the Virginia statute legalizing forced sterilizations of so-called "mentally deficient" wards of the state was unconstitutional. Buck, a young woman whose mother was also committed and whose daughter was deemed to be "not quite normal" was declared by Justice Oliver Wendell Holmes in his decision to be "unfit" to "continue her kind." His pronouncement that "three generations of imbeciles is enough" was used as the rallying cry for eugenicists who saw to it that more than 60,000 forcible sterilizations were performed on those considered "genetically unfit." Imparato and Sommers say that while such practices are condemned, several well-respected individuals, including the embryologist Bob Edwards and the bioethicist Peter Singer and professional bodies such as the American College of Obstetrics and Gynecologists, have made remarks that show they view people with disabilities as somehow less than those who do not bear such a "burden." These researchers and groups talk about the "quality" of children and see children with disabilities as "draining limited resources." In contrast to this, the authors point to the United Nations's Convention on the Rights of the Persons with Disabilities and the Americans with Disabilities Act, which recognize disability as a natural part of the human experience that should not limit one's full participation in society. They maintain that talking about "good genes" and "bad genes" and valuing some lives over others are violations of human rights.*

In its preamble, the recently unveiled U.N. Convention on the Rights of Persons With Disabilities recognizes "the inherent dignity and worth and equal and inalienable rights of all members of the human family as the foundation of freedom, justice and peace in the world."

We wonder what Oliver Wendell Holmes would have said about that.

This month [May 2007] marked the 80th anniversary of the disgraceful Supreme Court decision in *Buck v. Bell*, which upheld Virginia's involuntary sterilization laws. In his majority opinion, Holmes declared: "It is better for all the world, if instead of waiting to execute degenerate offspring for crime, or to let them starve for their imbecility, society can prevent those who are manifestly unfit from continuing their kind . . . Three generations of imbeciles is enough."

Although eugenics was eventually dismissed as "junk science," it didn't happen before states authorized more than 60,000 forcible sterilizations and segregated, institutionalized, and denied marriage and parental rights to those deemed "genetically unfit."

Contemporary Echoes

Though society may be inclined to regard Holmes's detestable opinion in *Buck v. Bell* as a relic of a time past, eerie similarities exist in contemporary remarks of the well-respected.

Justifying the sterilization of "genetically unfit" individuals, Holmes wrote that Carrie Buck was "the probable potential parent of socially inadequate offspring."

Some 72 years later, renowned embryologist Bob Edwards said, "Soon it will be a sin for parents to have a child that carries the heavy burden of genetic disease. We are entering a world where we have to consider the quality of our children."

Not long ago, an embryo entrepreneur boasted on her business's Web site, "In the process of screening donors, we select only those that have clean medical backgrounds. . . . The embryos that are available have all been medically 'graded,' so that the recipient family knows the quality of the embryos that they will be implanting."

In the past, eugenicists emphasized the "burden" of disability. Holmes wrote that individuals with disabilities "sap the strength of the State."

In recent years, Peter Singer, a professor of bioethics at Princeton University, has said, "It does not seem quite wise to increase any further draining of limited resources by increasing the number of children with impairments."

In January, the American College of Obstetricians and Gynecologists urged all women regardless of age to undergo prenatal screening for Down syndrome, aware of statistics that greater than 85 percent of pregnancies diagnosed with Down syndrome end in abortion.

Several states recognize life with a disability as an injury in "wrongful life" lawsuits, and certain judges who hear these cases agree that in some instances, selective abortions help answer a greater policy concern in curbing health-care expenditures.

[In late 2006], Britain's Royal College of Obstetricians and Gynecologists argued for "active euthanasia" of significantly disabled newborns to spare parents emotional and financial burden.

Two years earlier, the Groningen Protocol emerged in the Netherlands; it proposed selection criteria for euthanizing babies and children with disabilities.

And across the United States, "futile care" policies have required that the most vulnerable give up their hospital beds—and lives—for those with more "potential."

A Natural Part of Human Existence

In stark contrast to words such as "defective," "burdensome" and "futile" are the words of civil rights laws that liberate and defend.

The Americans With Disabilities Act recognizes disability as a natural part of the human experience that in no way should limit an individual's ability to participate fully in all aspects of society. The U.N. convention reaffirms that people with disabilities have both a right to life and a right to the effective enjoyment of that life on an equal basis with others.

On this 80th anniversary of *Buck*, let's not foolishly believe that victims of eugenics are an artifact of history. So long as we speak in terms of good genes and bad genes, recognize a life with a disability as an injury, and allow health policies to value some lives over others, we continue to create human rights violations every day.

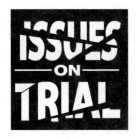

CHAPTER 2

Defining Free and Appropriate Education for Children of All Abilities

Case Overview

Hendrick Hudson School District v. Rowley (1982)

Before 1975 children with disabilities were largely excluded from public education. In 1975 Congress enacted the Education for All Handicapped Children Act (EAHCA or EHA). The EHA required that public schools accepting federal funds provide equal access to "free appropriate public education" for children with physical and mental disabilities. Schools were required to create an individualized education program (IEP) for each student, establish procedures allowing parents to participate in its formulation, and dispute the final plan. In 1982 *Hendrick Hudson School District v. Rowley* provided an opportunity for the U.S. Supreme Court to clarify the intent and application of the EHA.

The plaintiff, Amy Rowley, was a substantially deaf first-grader. Though none challenged her right to attend public school, parents and school officials disagreed on the level of support she required. According to her IEP, Amy was to be placed with typical students, use an amplification system, and receive instruction from a tutor an hour a day and from a speech therapist three hours a week. This support, however, gave her access to only about half the information available to other students. Amy's parents argued that she should also be provided with an in-class sign-language interpreter to remedy the imbalance. School officials disagreed, arguing that Amy performed in the top half of her class and was thus receiving sufficient assistance.

Amy's parents requested an impartial hearing after their request for an interpreter was denied. The examiner agreed with school officials. Amy's parents challenged the decision in New York's federal district court. Judge Vincent L. Broderick considered three interpretations of "appropriate education." It could mean an "adequate education" (passing from grade to grade), an education that allowed children to reach their full potential, or an education that provided benefits "commensurate with the opportunity provided other children." Broderick adopted the third interpretation, and the court sided with the Rowleys. The U.S. Court of Appeals for the Second Circuit affirmed the district court's decision. The U.S. Supreme Court, however, reversed the judgment.

Writing for the majority, William Rehnquist argued that the primary intent of the EHA was to end the practice of excluding children with disabilities from public education. While schools must provide a "basic floor of opportunity," he wrote, they need not provide equal opportunity for learning. Rehnquist also highlighted the procedural requirements of the EHA: "It seems to us no exaggeration to say that Congress placed . . . as much emphasis upon compliance with procedures giving parents and guardians a large measure of participation at every stage of the administrative process as it did upon the measurement of the resulting IEP against a substantive standard." School officials were judged as complying with the EHA, since they had opened their doors to Amy, developed a beneficial IEP, and allowed parental participation throughout.

In his dissent, Byron White argued that Congress's intent was to provide equal educational opportunity and that the package of services provided to Amy did not accomplish this. It is hardly equal opportunity, he argued, if Amy had access to only half of what was said in the classroom.

Rowley stands as the primary precedent used when determining whether school districts are providing appropriate education for children with disabilities. The merits of *Rowley* have been debated, however. Though widely recognized for upholding disability rights, it has been criticized for setting the bar too low, for relying too heavily on procedural protections, and for leaving too much to the discretion of the states. In 1990 the EHA was reauthorized as the Individuals with Disabilities Education Act (IDEA), which imposes higher standards for what constitutes a free, appropriate public education.

> *"To require ... the furnishing of every
> special service necessary to maximize
> each handicapped child's potential is,
> we think, further than Congress in-
> tended to go."*

Majority Opinion: Free and Appropriate Education Does Not Include Every Special Service

William Rehnquist

William Rehnquist was nominated by President Richard Nixon to the Supreme Court in 1971. After serving as associate justice for fifteen years, he was nominated in 1986 by President Ronald Reagan to be chief justice of the United States. In his written opinion in Hendrick Hudson School District v. Rowley *(1982), the first special-education case to come before the Supreme Court, Rehnquist explains why the Hendrick Hudson School District was not required to provide Amy Rowley, a deaf fourth-grader, with a sign-language interpreter in her classroom. The case had been filed by Rowley's parents, who argued that while the special education services she was receiving (including a hearing aid, daily tutoring, and instruction from a speech therapist) were helping their daughter advance (she was in the top half of her class), she was not performing as well academically as she would if she were hearing. They argued, and the lower courts agreed, that Rowley was not receiving the "free and appropriate education" guaranteed by the Education for All Handicapped Children*

William Rehnquist, majority opinion, *Hendrick Hudson School District v. Rowley*, U.S. Supreme Court, 1982.

Act (EAHCA or EHA) because she was not being given the opportunity to reach her full potential. In his opinion, Rehnquist denied the Rowleys' petition, saying that local school districts are not obliged to provide services that such children need to reach their "full academic potential" but rather entitles children with disabilities to a public education from which they can derive "some educational benefit." Reviewing the congressional history and legislative intent of the EAHCA, he said, shows that Congress enacted the law with the clear recognition that too many children with disabilities had been denied educational opportunities. The EAHCA sought to remedy the problem of children with special needs being excluded from public schools and intended to open the door to a "basic floor of opportunity," which "consists of access to specialized instruction and related services which are individually designed to provide educational benefit to the handicapped child." According to Rehnquist, a special education for a child with a disability should deliver some degree of benefit, but a school's obligation under the EAHCA was satisfied by providing benefit that satisfied the minimum, rather than the maximum extent possible.

This case arose in connection with the education of Amy Rowley, a deaf student at the Furnace Woods School in the Hendrick Hudson Central School District, Peekskill, N.Y. Amy has minimal residual hearing and is an excellent lip-reader. During the year before she began attending Furnace Woods, a meeting between her parents and school administrators resulted in a decision to place her in a regular kindergarten class in order to determine what supplemental services would be necessary to her education. Several members of the school administration prepared for Amy's arrival by attending a course in sign-language interpretation, and a teletype machine was installed in the principal's office to facilitate communication with her parents who are also deaf. At the end of the trial period it was determined that Amy should remain in the kindergarten class, but that she should be provided with an FM hearing aid which would amplify words spoken into a wireless receiver by the teacher or fellow students during certain classroom activities. Amy successfully completed her kindergarten year.

As required by the [Education for All Handicapped Children] Act, an IEP [individualized education program] was prepared for Amy during the fall of her first-grade year. The IEP provided that Amy should be educated in a regular classroom at Furnace Woods, should continue to use the FM hearing aid, and should receive instruction from a tutor for the deaf for one hour each day and from a speech therapist for three hours each week. The Rowleys agreed with the IEP but insisted that Amy also be provided a qualified sign-language interpreter in all of her academic classes. Such an interpreter had been placed in Amy's kindergarten class for a two-week experimental period, but the interpreter had reported that Amy did not need his services at that time. The school administrators likewise concluded that Amy did not need such an interpreter in her first-grade classroom. They reached this conclusion after consulting the school district's Committee on the Handicapped, which had received expert evidence from Amy's parents on the importance of a sign-language interpreter, received testimony from Amy's teacher and other persons familiar with her academic and social progress, and visited a class for the deaf.

When their request for an interpreter was denied, the Rowleys demanded and received a hearing before an independent examiner. After receiving evidence from both sides, the examiner agreed with the administrators' determination that an interpreter was not necessary because "Amy was achieving educationally, academically, and socially" without such assistance. The examiner's decision was affirmed on appeal by the New York Commissioner of Education on the basis of substantial evidence in the record. . . .

The District Court found that Amy "is a remarkably well adjusted child" who interacts and communicates well with her classmates and has "developed an extraordinary rapport" with her teachers. It also found that "she performs better than the average child in her class and is advancing easily from grade to grade," but "that she understands considerably less of what goes on in class than she would if she were not deaf" and thus "is not learning as much, or performing as well academically, as she would without her handicap." This disparity between Amy's achievement and her potential led the court to decide that she was not receiving a "free appropriate public education" which the court defined as "an opportunity to achieve [her] full potential commensurate with the opportunity provided to other children." According to the District Court, such a standard "requires that the potential of the handicapped child be measured and compared to his or her performance, and that the remaining differential or 'shortfall' be compared to the shortfall experienced by nonhandicapped children." The District Court's definition arose from its assumption that the responsibility for "giv[ing] content to the requirement of an 'appropriate education,'" had "been left entirely to the [federal] courts and the hearing officers."

A divided panel of the United States Court of Appeals for the Second Circuit affirmed. The Court of Appeals "agree[d] with the [D]istrict [C]ourt's conclusions of law," and held that its "findings of fact [were] not clearly erroneous." ...

Interpreting the EAHCA

This is the first case in which this Court has been called upon to interpret any provision of the [EAHCA]. As noted previously, the District Court and Court of Appeals concluded that "the Act itself does nor define 'appropriate education.'" ...

We are loath to conclude that Congress failed to offer any assistance in defining the meaning of the principal substantive phrase used in the Act. It is beyond dispute that, contrary to the conclusions of the courts below, the Act does expressly define "free appropriate public education":

> The term "free appropriate public education" means special education and related services which (A) have been provided at public expenses, under public supervision and direction, and without charge, (B) meet the standards of the State educational agency, (C) include an appropriate preschool, elementary, or secondary school education in the State involved, and (D) are provided in conformity with the individualized education program. . . .
>
> "Special education," as referred to in this definition, means "specially designed instruction, at no cost to parents or guardians, to meet the unique needs of a handicapped child, including classroom instruction, instruction in physical education, home instruction, and instruction in hospitals and institutions." "Related services" are defined as "transportation, and such developmental, corrective, and other supportive services . . . as may be required to assist a handicapped child to benefit from special education." . . .

According to the definitions contained in the Act, a "free appropriate public education" consists of educational instruction specially designed to meet the unique needs of the handicapped child, supported by such services as are necessary to permit the child "to benefit" from the instruction. Almost as a checklist for adequacy under the Act, the definition also requires that such instruction and services be provided at public expense and under public supervision, meet the State's educational standards, approximate the grade levels used in the State's regular education, and comport with the child's IEP. Thus, if personalized instruction is being provided with sufficient supportive services to permit the child to benefit from the instruction, and the other items on the definitional checklist are satisfied, the child is receiving a "free appropriate public education" as defined by the Act. . . .

Noticeably absent from the language of the statute is any substantive standard prescribing of the level of education to be accorded handicapped children. Certainly the language of the statute contains no requirement like the one imposed by the lower courts—that States maximize the potential of handicapped children "commensurate with the opportunity provided to other children." . . .

Intent of the Act

By passing the Act, Congress sought primarily to make public education available to handicapped children. But in seeking to provide such access to public education, Congress did not impose upon the states any greater substantive educational standard than would be necessary to make such access meaningful. Indeed, Congress expressly "recognized that in many instances the process of providing special education and related services to handicapped children is not guaranteed to produce any particular outcome." Thus, the intent of the Act was more to open the door of public education to handicapped children on appropriate terms than to guarantee any particular level of education once inside. . . .

That the Act imposes no clear obligation upon recipient States beyond the requirement that handicapped children receive some form of specialized education is perhaps best demonstrated by the fact that Congress, in explaining the need for the Act, equated an "appropriate education" to the receipt of some specialized educational services. The Senate report states: '[T]he most recent statistics provided by the Bureau of Education for the Handicapped estimate that of the more than 8 million children . . . with handicapping conditions requiring special education and related services, only 3.9 million such children are "receiving an appropriate education." . . .

It is evident from the legislative history that the characterization of handicapped children as "served" referred to children who were receiving some form of specialized educational services from the States, and that the characterization of children as "unserved" referred to those who were receiving no specialized educational services. For example, a letter sent to the United States Commissioner of Education by the House Committee on Education and Labor, signed by two key sponsors of the Act in the House, asked the commissioner to identify the number of handicapped "children served" in each State. The letter asked for statistics on the number of children "being served" in various types of "special education program[s]" and the number of children who were not "receiving educational services." . . .

Not Required to Maximize Potential

Respondents contend that "the goal of the Act is to provide each handicapped child with an equal educational opportunity." We think, however, that the requirement that a State provide specialized educational services to handicapped children generates no additional requirement that the services so provided be sufficient to maximize each child's potential "commensurate with the opportunity provided other children." . . .

The educational opportunities provided by our public school systems undoubtedly differ from student to student, depending upon a myriad of factors that might affect a particular student's ability to assimilate information presented in the classroom. The requirement that States provide "equal" educational opportunities would thus seem to present an entirely unworkable standard requiring impossible measurements and comparisons. Similarly, furnishing handicapped children with only such services as are available to nonhandicapped children would in all probability fall short of the statutory requirement of "free appropriate public education"; to require, on the other hand, the furnishing of every special service necessary to maximize each handicapped child's potential is, we think, further than Congress intended to go. Thus to speak in terms of "equal" services in one instance gives less than what is required by the Act and in another instance more. The theme of the Act is "free appropriate public education," a phrase which is too complex to be captured by the word "equal" whether one is speaking of opportunities or services. . . .

The District Court and the Court of Appeals thus erred when they held that the Act requires New York to maximize the potential of each handicapped child commensurate with the opportunity provided nonhandicapped children. Desirable though that goal might be, it is not the standard that Congress imposed upon States which receive funding under the Act. Rather, Congress sought primarily to identify and evaluate handicapped children, and to provide them with access to a free public education.

A Basic Floor of Opportunity

Implicit in the congressional purpose of providing access to a "free appropriate public education" is the requirement that the education to which access is provided be sufficient to confer some educational benefit upon the handicapped child. It would do little good for Congress to spend millions of dollars in providing access to public education only to have the handicapped child receive no benefit from that education. The statutory definition of "free appropriate public education," in addition to requiring that States provide each child with "specially designed instruction," expressly requires the provision of "such . . . supportive services . . . as may be required to assist a handicapped child to benefit from special education." We therefore conclude that the "basic floor of opportunity" provided by the Act consists of access to specialized instruction and related services which are individually designed to provide educational benefit to the handicapped child.

The determination of when handicapped children are receiving sufficient educational benefits to satisfy the requirements of the Act presents a more difficult problem. The Act requires participating States to educate a wide spectrum of handicapped children, from the marginally hearing-impaired to the profoundly retarded and palsied. It is clear that the benefits obtainable by children at one end of the spectrum will differ dramatically from those obtainable by children at the other end, with infinite variations in between. One child may have little difficulty competing successfully in an academic setting with nonhandicapped children while another child may encounter great difficulty in acquiring even the most basic of self-maintenance skills. We do not attempt today to establish any one test for determining the adequacy of educational benefits conferred upon all children covered by the Act. Because in this case we are presented with a handicapped child who is receiving substantial specialized instruction and related services, and who is performing above average in the regular classrooms of a public school system, we confine our analysis to that situation.

The Act requires participating States to educate handicapped children with nonhandicapped children whenever possible. When that "mainstreaming" preference of the Act has been met and a child is being educated in the regular classrooms of a public school system, the system itself monitors the educational progress of the child. Regular examinations are administered, grades are awarded, and yearly advancement to higher grade levels is permitted for those children who attain an adequate knowledge of the course material. The grading and advancement system thus constitutes an important factor in determining educational benefit. Children who graduate from our public school systems are considered by our society to have been "educated" at least to the grade level they have completed, and access to an "education" for handicapped children is precisely what Congress sought to provide in the Act.

When the language of the Act and its legislative history are considered together, the requirements imposed by Congress become tolerably clear. Insofar as a State is required to provide a handicapped child with a "free appropriate public education," we hold that it satisfies this requirements by providing personalized instruction with sufficient support services to permit the child to benefit educationally from that instruction. Such instruction and services must be provided at public expense, must meet the State's educational standards, must approximate the grade levels used in the State's regular education, and must comport with the child's IEP. In addition, the IEP, and therefore the personalized instruction, should be formulated in accordance with the requirements of the Act, and if the child is being educated in the regular classrooms of the public education system, should be reasonably calculated to enable the child to achieve passing marks and advance from grade to grade. . . .

Procedural Safeguards

The parties disagree sharply over the meaning of these provisions, petitioners contending that courts are given only limited authority to review for state compliance with the Act's procedural requirements and no power to review the substance of the state program, and respondents contending that the Act requires courts to exercise de novo [literally, "anew"] review over state educational decisions and policies. We find petitioners' contention unpersuasive, for Congress expressly rejected provisions that would have so severely restricted the role of reviewing courts. In substituting the current language of the statute for language that would have made state administrative findings conclusive if supported by substantial evidence, the Conference Committee explained that courts were to make "independent decisions based on a preponderance of the evidence."

But although we find that this grant of authority is broader than claimed by petitioners, we think the fact that it is found in 1415 of the Act, which is entitled "Procedural Safeguards," is not without significance. When the elaborate and highly specific procedural safeguards embodied in [section] 1415 are contrasted with the general and somewhat imprecise substantive admonitions contained in the Act, we think that the importance Congress attached to these procedural safeguards cannot be gainsaid. It seems to us no exaggeration to say that Congress placed every bit as much emphasis upon compliance with procedures giving parents and guardians a large measure of participation at every stage of the administrative process, as it did upon the measurement of the resulting IEP against a substantive standard. We think that the congressional emphasis upon full participation of concerned parties throughout the development of the IEP, as well as the requirements that state and local plans be submitted to the Secretary for approval, demonstrate the legislative conviction that adequate compliance with the procedures prescribed would in most cases assure much if not all of what Congress wished in the way of substantive content in an IEP.

Thus, the provision that a reviewing court base its decision on the "preponderance of the evidence" is by no means an invitation to the court to substitute their own notions of sound educational policy for those of the school authorities which they review. The very importance which Congress has attached to compliance with certain procedures in the preparation of an IEP would be frustrated if a court were permitted simply to set state decisions at nought. The fact that 1415(e) requires that the reviewing court "receive the records of the [state] administrative proceedings" carries with it the implied requirement that due weight shall be given to these proceedings. And we find nothing in the Act to suggest that merely because Congress was rather sketchy in establishing substantive requirements, as opposed to procedural requirements for the preparation of an IEP, it intended that reviewing courts should have a free hand to impose substantive standards of review which cannot be derived from the Act itself. In short, the statutory authorization to grant "such relief as the court determines is appropriate" cannot be read without reference to the obligations, largely procedural in nature, which are imposed upon recipient States by Congress.

Therefore, a court's inquiry in suits brought under 1415(e)(2) is twofold. First, has the State complied with the procedures set forth in the Act? And second, is the individualized educational program developed through the Act's procedures reasonably calculated to enable the child to receive educational benefits? If these requirements are met, the State has complied with the obligations imposed by Congress and the courts can require no more.

In assuring that the requirements of the Act have been met, courts must be careful to avoid imposing their view of preferable educational methods upon the States. The primary responsibility for formulating the education to be accorded a handicapped child, and for choosing the educational method most suitable to the child's needs, was left by the Act to state and local educational agencies in cooperation with the parents or guardian of the child. . . .

Applying these principles to the facts of this case, we conclude that the court of Appeals erred in affirming the decision of the District Court. Neither the District Court nor the Court of Appeals found that petitioners had failed to comply with the procedures of the Act, and the findings of neither court would support a conclusion that Amy's educational program failed to comply with the substantive requirements of the Act. On the contrary, the District Court found that the "evidence firmly establishes that Amy is receiving an 'adequate' education, since she performs better than the average child in her class and is advancing easily from grade to grade." In light of this finding, and of the fact that Amy was receiving personalized instruction and related services calculated by the Furnace Woods school administrators to meet her educational needs, the lower courts should not have concluded that the Act requires the provision of a sign-language interpreter. Accordingly, the decision of the Court of appeals is reversed and the case is remanded for further proceedings consistent with this opinion.

"Amy Rowley, without a sign-language
interpreter, comprehends less than half
of what is said in the classroom—less
than half of what normal children comprehend. This is hardly an equal opportunity to learn, even if Amy makes
passing grades."

Dissenting Opinion: Every Child Should Have an Equal Opportunity to Learn

Byron Raymond White

Appointed to the court by President John F. Kennedy in 1962, Byron Raymond White served as an associate justice on the Supreme Court until his retirement in 1993. White, along with Justices William J. Brennan and Thurgood Marshall, dissented in the case of Hendrick Hudson School District v. Rowley, *in which the Court denied the petition of the parents of a deaf fourth-grader who sought to obtain special services for her at school. Amy Rowley was performing well in school and received some special education services, but she was not achieving her full potential because, without an interpreter, she could not understand half of what was said in her lessons. The Supreme Court denied her claim, saying that the school district had provided her with the minimum of what they were required to provide under the Education for All Handicapped Children Act (EAHCA or EHA). In the following dissenting opinion White counters this notion, arguing that the standard adopted by the*

Byron Raymond White, dissenting opinion, *Hendrick Hudson School District v. Rowley,*
U.S. Supreme Court, 1982.

majority in the decision ignores the intent of Congress to provide a "full educational opportunity to all handicapped children." He says that the conclusion that the law was satisfied if the child received "some benefit" from the educational program falls far short of what the act intended. According to White, Congress meant the Act to "eliminate the effects of the handicap, at least to the extent that the child will be given an equal opportunity to learn if that is reasonably possible," a standard that could not be satisfied by demonstrating that the child was receiving passing grades.

In order to reach its result in this case, the majority opinion contradicts itself, the language of the statute, and the legislative history. Both the majority's standard for a "free appropriate education" and its standard for judicial review disregard congressional intent.

The Act Intended to Provide More

The majority first turns its attention to the meaning of a "free appropriate public education." The [Education for All Handicapped Children Act] provides:

> The term 'free appropriate public education' means special education and related services which (A) have been provided at public expense, under public supervision and direction, and without charge, (B) meet the standard of the State educational agency, (C) include an appropriate preschool, elementary, or secondary school education in the State involved, and (D) are provided in conformity with the individualized education program required under section 1414(a)(5) of this title.

The majority reads this statutory language as establishing a congressional intent limited to bringing "previously excluded handicapped children into the public education systems of the States and [requiring] the States to adopt procedures which would result in individualized consideration of and instruction for each child." In its attempt to constrict the definition of "appropriate" and the thrust of the Act, the majority opinion states: "Noticeably absent from the language of the statute is any substantive standard prescribing the level of education to be accorded handicapped children. Certainly the language of the statute contains no requirement like the one imposed by the lower courts—that States maximize the potential of handicapped children 'commensurate with the opportunity provided to other children.'" . . .

The majority opinion announces a different substantive standard, that "Congress did not impose upon the States any greater substantive standard than would be necessary to make such access meaningful." While "meaningful" is no more enlightening than "appropriate," the Court purports to clarify itself. Because Amy was provided with some specialized instruction from which she obtained some benefit and because she passed from grade to grade, she was receiving a meaningful and therefore appropriate education.

This falls far short of what the Act intended. The Act details as specifically as possible the kind of specialized education each handicapped child must receive. It would apparently satisfy the Court's standard of "access to specialized instruction and related services which are individually designed to provide educational benefit to the handicapped child," for a deaf child such as Amy to be given a teacher with a loud voice, for she would benefit from that service. The Act requires more. It defines "special education" to mean "specifically designed instruction, at no cost to parents or guardians, to meet the unique needs of a handicapped child. . . ." Providing a teacher with a loud voice would not meet Amy's needs and would not satisfy the Act. The basic floor of opportunity is instead, as the courts below recognized, intended to eliminate the effects of the handicap, at least to the extent that the child will be given an equal opportunity to learn if that is reasonably possible. Amy Rowley, without a sign-language interpreter, comprehends less than half of what is said in the class-room—less than half of what normal children comprehend. This is hardly an equal opportunity to learn, even if Amy makes passing grades. . . .

A More Searching Inquiry

The Court's discussion of the standard for judicial review is as flawed as its discussion of a "free appropriate public educa-tion." According to the Court, a court can ask only whether the State has "complied with the procedures set forth in the Act" and whether the individualized education program is "reasonably calculated to enable the child to receive educa-tional benefits." Both the language of the Act and the legisla-tive history, however, demonstrate that Congress intended the courts to conduct a far more searching inquiry. . . .

The legislative history shows that judicial review is not limited to procedural matters and that the state educational agencies are given first, but not final, responsibility for the content of a handicapped child's education. The Conference committee directs courts to make an "independent decision." The deliberate change in the review provision is an unusually clear indication that Congress intended courts to undertake substantive review instead of relying on the conclusions of the state agency. . . .

Thus, the Court's limitations on judicial review have no support in either the language of the Act or the legislative his-tory. Congress did not envision that inquiry would end if a showing is made that the child is receiving passing marks and is advancing from grade to grade. Instead, it intended to per-mit a full and searching inquiry into any aspect of a handi-capped child's education. The Court's standard, for example, would not permit a challenge to part of the IEP; the legislative history demonstrate beyond doubt that Congress intended such challenge to be possible, even if the plan as developed is reasonably calculated to give the child some benefits.

Rowley Was a Revolutionary Development for People with Disabilities

Paul F. Stavis

*Paul F. Stavis is director of the Bureau of House Counsel, New
York State Department of Health, and is an adjunct professor of
law and psychiatry at the Albany Law School. In the following
essay he offers an analysis of* Hendrick Hudson School District
v. Rowley. *He first presents the facts of the case, explaining that
the case involved the education plan of Amy Rowley, a deaf
fourth-grader whose parents argued that her school district
should provide her with a sign-language interpreter so that she
may reach her full academic potential. The Supreme Court denied the Rowleys' request, saying that the Education for All
Handicapped Children Act (EAHCA or EHA) was not intended
to provide children with disabilities every service but rather a
"basic floor" of opportunity for education. Stavis describes the
dissent in the case, written by Byron Raymond White, who argues that the act guaranteed an "equal educational opportunity,"
which Rowley was being denied because she could not hear the
class proceedings. The disagreement between the Supreme Court
justices, according to Stavis, comes down to their differences on*

Paul F. Stavis, "Free Appropriate Education—The Supreme Court's First Decision,"
Quality of Care Newsletter, no. 12, July–August 1982. Reproduced by permission.

whether the EAHCA mandates minimum or maximum educa-tional services for children with disabilities. The majority saw the act as intending to ameliorate the plight of the many chil-dren who had no access to education, while the minority be-lieved that the act was intended to mandate that states provide maximum opportunities to children with disabilities equal to those of their peers. Stavis notes that the decision left much to the states but says that even if advocates for children with dis-abilities are disappointed with the ruling, the decision was a vic-tory because it read into the law new substantial rights and pro-tections for children with disabilities and opened the door to public education to them.

The United States Supreme Court recently decided a case having significant impact on the education of all children with handicapping conditions. This case is *Hendrick Hudson School District v. Rowley*, decided by the Court on June 28, 1982. The Court agreed to decide the question of whether a sign language interpreter was necessary in order to provide Amy Rowley, a deaf student, with a free appropriate education as required under the Federal Education for all Handicapped Children Act of 1975. This is the first case the Supreme Court has entertained concerning legal issues arising out of this im-portant law which guarantees a "free appropriate education" to all children with disabilities. Two questions were specifically addressed: First, what is the practical meaning of the statute's term "appropriate education", and second, what is the role of the state and federal courts in exercising the judicial review granted under this law.

The plaintiff, Amy Rowley, is a deaf student with minimal residual hearing but with an excellent ability to lip-read. An Individual Education Plan (IEP) was prepared for Amy during the fall of her first grade year which provided that she should be educated in a regular classroom with non-handicapped students at the Furnace Woods School in Peekskill, New York. The IEP also required that Amy make use of a hearing aid and receive instruction from a tutor for the deaf for one hour each day and from a speech therapist three hours each week. In order to further assist Amy, several school administrators also attended a course in sign-language interpretation and a teletype machine was installed to facilitate communication with Amy's parents who are also deaf.

However, despite these specialized services, Amy's parents disagreed with the IEP because it did not require that Amy be provided with an in-class sign language interpreter because, while Amy performed in the top half of her class without an interpreter, she nevertheless missed a substantial portion of what was said in class. Her parents strongly believed she was entitled to assistance in obtaining full comprehension in the classroom so as to have an equal opportunity for maximum achievement as other non-handicapped children. Such an interpreter was placed in Amy's kindergarten class for a two-week experimental period, but the interpreter reported that his services were not really needed. The school administrators then concluded that none should be provided, and the school district's Committee on the Handicapped agreed.

Since P.L. 94-142 provides a specific due process procedure to resolve such disagreements, Amy's parents requested and received an impartial hearing after their request for an interpreter for Amy was denied. The impartial hearing examiner agreed with the school district's Committee on the Handicapped and other teachers familiar with Amy's progress that an interpreter was not needed. The Commissioner of Education affirmed this decision upon administrative appeal.

Subsequently, the Rowleys brought an action in the Federal District Court in New York to challenge the decision denying Amy the services of an interpreter. The Court ruled that Amy was not receiving all the services of a full appropriate education because she was not being provided "an opportunity to achieve (her) full potential commensurate with the opportunity provided to other children." A divided panel of the

U.S. Court of Appeals for the Second Circuit agreed and affirmed the district court's decision saying that the Act did not define the term "appropriate education," leaving that decision "to the courts and hearing officers."

Majority Opinion: Two Clear Rights

The United States Supreme Court agreed to review this case and concluded in its decision that Public Law 94-142, although "cryptic" in parts, nonetheless mandates two clear rights for handicapped children:

1. a "free appropriate public education," meaning special educational and related services at public expense (i.e., without charge), meeting the standards of approximate grade levels of the State education agency within the context of an individualized education program written with parental participation; and

2. due process, including access to judicial review to determine that the State has complied with the Act and that the written individualized educational program is "reasonably calculated to enable the child to receive educational benefits," e.g. achieving passing marks and grade advancement.

With this reasoning, the Supreme Court decided that Amy Rowley was not entitled to have a sign-language interpreter. The officials of the school district and Committee on the Handicapped complied with all procedures of the Act and in doing so, composed an individual educational program reasonably calculated to allow Amy a free and appropriate education. Moreover, the facts show that Amy was doing very well, indeed above average, in her class and was advancing easily from grade to grade. In short, her program was working. Given this procedural compliance and a reasonable individualized program, the Supreme Court held it was improper for the District Court and Circuit Court of Appeals to substitute their judgment for the duly constituted State education program.

The Dissent: The Act Affords More

The legal viewpoint of the dissenting opinion by Justice [Byron Raymond] White, joined by Justices [Thurgood] Marshall and [William] Brennan, sharply contrasts the majority position of mandating courts to defer to the reasonable actions of the State education system. The dissent agreed that the Act does not expressly contain a substantive standard for an "appropriate education," however, merely receiving passing marks and grades was not all that it affords handicapped children. The dissent emphasized a Senate report stating that the Act guaranteed an "equal educational opportunity" and that, in Amy's case, she was missing half of class proceedings without an interpreter. Therefore, the dissent thought that this was not a situation which gave Amy an opportunity commensurate with non-handicapped students. The dissent also would give greater discretion to the courts to scrutinize individual educational programs beyond their compliance with a mere standard of being "reasonably calculated" to produce educational benefits.

Maximum vs. Minimum Services

Put in simpler terms, the disagreement between the majority and dissent is one of maximum versus minimum mandated services under the Education for all Handicapped Children Act. The majority saw this law and its legislative history as ameliorating the plight of as many as 1.7 million handicapped children not receiving any education at all and 2.5 million not receiving an appropriate one. In other words, the law was to be a minimum "floor of opportunity" for a federally established foundation upon which states could build education programs for handicapped children consonant with the philosophy of the individual state educational system.

The dissent believed that this law was intended to mandate that states provide maximum opportunities for handicapped children to equal those of non-handicapped students. The dissent also focused more on the available opportunities and services and less than the majority upon the particular performances of the individual student, i.e., Amy was doing better-than average in school.

The *Rowley* decision follows traditional federalist constitutional construction in allowing the federal government to prescribe minimum standards for state activities, and allowing the states to do more if they wish. Education has been historically within the province of the states, with the first major federal intrusion being the landmark *Brown v. Board of Education*, which ordered public schools desegregated. In *Rowley*, the Supreme Court was faithful in declaring newly created federal statutory rights for handicapped children, while not having it seem that the federal bureaucracy and judiciary would usurp this primary state function. It also expressed concern that the multiplicity of state educational philosophies and experimental approaches would be homogenized if the federal influence for uniformity was too strong. Again, traditionally the states have been allowed to adopt different methods as long as they met minimum federal standards.

Understandably, the advocates for the handicapped generally favor the broader federal role expressed by the dissent. After all, many needed reforms for the handicapped, minorities and other disadvantaged have come from Washington, and have prevailed over state opposition in many instances. Yet, this decision was clearly a victory for handicapped children because the Supreme Court definitely read this law as providing new substantial rights and protections and, while not reading it as broadly as possible, this is a revolutionary development for handicapped children on a par with the *Brown* decision in that it now opens the public schoolhouse door to them.

> *"The 'some educational benefit' stan-*
> *dard no longer accurately reflects the*
> *requirements of the Individuals with*
> *Disabilities Education Act."*

Rowley's "Some Educational Benefit" Standard Does Not Reflect Current Requirements

Scott F. Johnson

Scott F. Johnson is a professor of law at Concord University School of Law and an adjunct professor of law at Franklin Pierce Law Center, where he teaches education-law courses. He has been counsel in a number of important special education cases and is the founder of NHEdLaw, LLC, and the Education Law Resource Center, which provide resources and information about education law topics to help parents, educators, and other professionals understand legal requirements and meet student needs. In the following essay, he views the Hendrick Hudson School District v. Rowley *ruling as the standard by which the notion of "free and appropriate public education" (FAPE) has been understood. In that case, brought by the parents of Amy Rowley, a deaf fourth-grader who was succeeding in school but not maximizing her potential, the plaintiffs argued that the school district ought to provide Rowley with a sign-language interpreter in her classroom to ensure she receive the education she was entitled to under the Education for All Handicapped Children Act (EAHCA or EHA). Rowley lost the case, with the Court finding that the act intended to provide a basic floor of education for children*

Scott F. Johnson, "Reexamining Rowley: A New Focus in Special Education Law," *The Beacon*, Fall 2003. Reproduced by permission.

with special needs and not to provide them with services to maximize their educational opportunities. Johnson argues that this "some educational benefit" standard in Rowley *no longer reflects the requirements of the Individuals with Disabilities Education Act (IDEA), which was the 1990 reauthorization of the EAHCA. Johnson says that new state standards and educational adequacy requirements provide the substantive requirements of FAPE, and these standards exceed the "some educational benefit" benchmark set by* Rowley. *He argues that this new view of* Rowley *requires a fundamental change in how courts, school districts, and parents should view special education services.*

The Individuals with Disabilities Education Act [IDEA] requires public schools to provide a Free, Appropriate Public Education (FAPE) to students with disabilities. Exactly what FAPE means or requires is an elusive topic.

Twenty years ago, in *Hendrick Hudson Central School District Board of Education v. Rowley*, the United States Supreme Court held that FAPE requires services that provide students with "some educational benefit." *Rowley* is undoubtedly the most important and influential case in special education law. The "some educational benefit" standard permeates nearly every aspect of special education because it is the standard against which services are measured. Subsequent courts have expanded on this "some educational benefit" requirement somewhat, but it remains essentially intact today.

Much has been written about *Rowley* and its impact in special education law. This paper presents a new and different perspective by exploring the *Rowley* standard for FAPE against the evolving backdrop of state educational standards and litigation about an adequate education under state constitutional law. Applying these standards to the analysis and reasoning in *Rowley*, this paper concludes that the "some educational benefit" standard no longer accurately reflects the requirements of the Individuals with Disabilities Education Act. Rather, state standards and educational adequacy requirements provide the substantive requirements of FAPE, and these standards exceed the "some educational benefit" benchmark. This conclusion requires a fundamental change in the way courts, school districts, and parents should view special education services. . . .

Evolving Standards of FAPE

The Individuals with Disabilities Education Act (IDEA) requires states and local school districts to provide students with disabilities with a "free and appropriate public education" (FAPE). FAPE is defined by the IDEA as special education and related services that:

(A) have been provided at public expense . . . without charge [to the parents];

(B) meet the standards of the State educational agency;

(C) include an appropriate preschool, elementary, or secondary school education in the State involved; and

(D) are provided in conformity with the student's individualized education program. . . .

While the statute defines FAPE, it does not describe the substantive requirements of FAPE, nor does it set any requisite standards or levels of learning achievement for students with disabilities. Because of this lack of substance, courts have struggled when asked to determine if a school district has provided a student with FAPE.

In *Board of Education of the Hendrick Hudson Central School District v. Rowley*, the United States Supreme Court attempted to determine the substantive standards of FAPE. The plaintiff in *Rowley* argued that FAPE required schools to maximize the potential of handicapped children commensurate with the opportunities provided to other children. The trial court agreed with this proportional maximization standard. The Court of Appeals affirmed the trial court's decision without much comment.

The Supreme Court overturned the Court of Appeals' decision, finding that the IDEA (then known as the EHA—Education Handicapped Act) did not require schools to proportionally maximize the potential of handicapped children. Rather, the Court said, Congress had more modest goals in mind. The Supreme Court relied upon the text and legislative history of the statute to find that Congressional intent was only to provide a "basic floor of opportunity" to students with disabilities by providing them access to public education, as opposed to addressing the quality of education received once in school. . . .

The Court determined, however, that some substantive standard for FAPE was "implicit in the congressional purpose of providing access to a free appropriate public education." The Court found that the substantive standard for FAPE required educational instruction specially designed to meet the unique needs of the handicapped child, supported by such services as are necessary to permit the child "to benefit" from the instruction.

The Court also noted that the statute provided a checklist of requirements for FAPE, including instruction at public expense and under public supervision, instruction that met the State's educational standards and approximated the grade levels used in the State's regular education system, and instruction that comported with the child's IEP. The Court concluded that "if personalized instruction is being provided with sufficient supportive services to permit the child to benefit from the instruction, and the other items on the definitional checklist are satisfied, the child is receiving a 'free appropriate public education' as defined by the Act."

The Court stated that when determining whether a student benefited from the services provided, "the achievement of passing marks and advancement from grade to grade will be one important factor in determining educational benefit," because passing grades and grade advancement were methods of monitoring educational progress for students being educated in regular classrooms.

Interpreting FAPE After *Rowley*

Subsequent court decisions interpreted *Rowley* to mean that the IDEA does not require schools to provide students with the best or optimal education, nor to ensure that students receive services to enable them to maximize their potential. Instead, schools are obligated only to offer services that provide students with "some educational benefit." Courts sometimes refer to this as the Cadillac versus Chevrolet argument, with the student entitled to a serviceable Chevrolet, not a Cadillac.

Some courts further refined the "some educational benefit" standard to require students to achieve "meaningful benefit" or to make "meaningful progress" in the areas where the student's disability affects their education. These courts held that while the IDEA does not require a school to maximize a student's potential, the student's potential and ability must be considered when determining whether he or she progressed and received educational benefit. Moreover, when a student displays considerable intellectual potential, the IDEA requires "a great deal more than a negligible benefit."

Despite a myriad of court decisions on the topic, school districts, parents, and courts still have little guidance on how to assess FAPE or educational benefit. In *Rowley*, the Supreme Court mentioned that grades and advancement from grade to grade were a factor in assessing benefit for mainstreamed students. Post-*Rowley* courts have viewed passing grades and grade advancement as important factors in determining if students received educational benefit. However, schools often modify grades for students with disabilities, so grades lose their validity as a measure of benefit or progress.

Some courts have looked at academic achievement testing, in addition to grades and grade advancement, to measure educational benefit. These courts relied upon "objective" standardized academic tests, such as performance on successive test scores, to measure educational benefit. Courts using this approach, however, produce varying results with similar information. The variance seems to be because courts do not have a substantive standard that defines what the student should know and be able to do at any given point in time. As a result, assessing benefit through improvement in test scores becomes a subjective analysis of whether gain of a certain amount on a particular test is sufficient progress.

The lack of substantive standards for FAPE combined the current Cadillac versus Chevrolet perspective facilitates a minimalist view of the substantive education that students with disabilities are entitled to receive and lowers expectations for students with disabilities. When Congress reauthorized the IDEA in 1997, it expressly noted that low expectations for students with disabilities had impeded implementation of the IDEA. Congress stated that educating students with disabilities could be more effective by "having high expectations for such children and ensuring their access in the general curriculum to the maximum extent possible."

Changes Affecting FAPE

Three important events occurred since the *Rowley* decision that impact the validity of the "some educational benefit" standard and change the nature of educational services that schools must provide to students who receive special education services under the IDEA.

The first event is state litigation over the constitutional requirements to provide an "adequate" education to students, including students with disabilities, under state constitutional law. An adequate education under state constitutional law requires the state to provide students with educational services targeted towards sufficient skills to be successful in society.

Some of these requirements are at odds with the *Rowley* "some educational benefit" standard and require a higher level of educational services.

The second event is the education standards movement that established high expectations for all students, including students with disabilities, through generally applicable content and proficiency standards. These standards define academic performance levels and provide specific substantive benchmarks that students should meet at specific points of their academic careers.

The third event occurred when Congress reauthorized the Individuals with Disabilities Act (IDEA) in 1997. At that time, Congress expressly changed the focus of the IDEA from access to education to high expectations and real educational results for children with disabilities. The 1997 changes emphasized that schools must provide students with disabilities with the same quality educational services already provided to students without disabilities, including access to a curriculum that incorporates state educational standards.

These changes require a reevaluation of what the standard for FAPE and *Rowley* mean today.

Adequate Education Under State Constitutional Law

Most states have state constitutional provisions requiring the state to provide educational services to students. Forty-four states have experienced litigation about the educational requirements outlined by their state constitutions. Most of these cases involved challenges to the state's system of financing education. Commentators organize school finance litigation into three "waves." Some contend that the last wave is ending and a potential fourth wave is beginning.

The first two waves of school finance litigation dealt primarily with equal protection or equity arguments surrounding school funding in local school districts. The third wave of school finance litigation focused on whether states have a constitutional obligation to provide students with a certain level or quality of education. This qualitative level of education is often referred to as "an adequate education."

Numerous state supreme courts held that their constitutions require their states to provide students with an adequate education. These court decisions create general state law educational standards and requirements. These standards are subsequently incorporated into the definition of FAPE for students with disabilities by the statutory provision that requires FAPE to "meet state standards" and include "an appropriate preschool, elementary, or secondary school education in the State involved." . . .

State constitutional mandates that require states to develop every child to his or her capacity and encourage each child to live up to his or her full human potential are directly at odds with the *Rowley* "basic floor of opportunity" standard. *Rowley* rejected the notion that the IDEA required states to maximize a student's potential. In a state where the state's constitution requires such a standard for all students, however, the requirement is incorporated into the IDEA's definition of FAPE as the standard for students with disabilities. Any other approach would run afoul of the IDEA's requirements.

Other state courts developed and applied similar constitutional requirements without express language regarding maximizing student potential, but these resulting standards remain clearly contrary to the minimalist guidelines set by *Rowley*. For example, the Kentucky Supreme Court decision in *Rose v. Council for Better Education* is one of the seminal cases about the requirements of an adequate education. In *Rose*, the court found the state was obligated to provide every child with:

> (i) [S]ufficient oral and written communication skills to enable students to function in a complex and rapidly changing civilization;

(ii) sufficient knowledge of economic, social, and political systems to enable the student to make informed choices;

(iii) sufficient understanding of governmental processes to enable the student to understand the issues that affect his or her community, state, and nation;

(iv) sufficient self-knowledge and knowledge of his or her mental and physical wellness;

(v) sufficient grounding in the arts to enable each student to appreciate his or her cultural and historical heritage;

(vi) sufficient training or preparation for advanced training in either academic or vocational fields so as to enable each child to choose and pursue life work intelligently; and

(vii) sufficient levels of academic or vocational skills to enable public school students to compete favorably with their counterparts in surrounding states, in academics or in the job market.

Several other state supreme courts adopted the seven criteria set forth in *Rose* as requirements under their state constitutions. These courts held that a constitutionally adequate education is not a minimal education. . . .

When states properly incorporate these constitutional requirements into the definition of FAPE, students with disabilities are entitled to more than just a "basic floor of opportunity" or "some educational benefit." These students are entitled to receive an education that allows for meaningful participation in a democratic society, and competition for post-secondary education and employment opportunities.

The IDEA requires incorporation of broad educational adequacy goals set forth in court decisions into Individual Educational Programs (IEPs) that meet the unique needs of each disabled student. Each student with a disability, as defined by the IDEA, is entitled to an IEP under the IDEA. The IEP must be tailored to meet the unique needs of the student. The IEP is the cornerstone of FAPE. Courts look at whether an IEP is appropriate when assessing whether a school district has provided FAPE. . . .

State Educational Standards

The definitional checklist of FAPE referenced by the Supreme Court in *Rowley* includes a requirement that the education provided to students with disabilities meet state standards. When the Court decided *Rowley*, this requirement did not have the same meaning it does today. At that time, most state standards did not involve substantive requirements for the educational services provided to students. Instead, standards addressed the process by which services would be provided.

However, since *Rowley*, educational standards have changed. Today, state and federal educational standards address the essential core of what students should know and be able to do. Known in the educational world as "standards-based education reform," state and federal educational standards now include content standards that specify what students should learn, proficiency standards that set expectations for what students must know and be able to do at specific times and assessment measures to determine if students have achieved these expectations.

Standards based education reform became prominent at the national level with Goals 2000. This federal law proposed national education goals and required states receiving funds under the program to develop strategies for meeting national education standards. These strategies, moreover, must include developing and adopting state education standards and assessment methods.

Other federal laws like Title I of the Elementary & Secondary Education Act [ESEA] (as amended by the Improving America's Schools Act of 1994) required states to develop or adopt challenging content, proficiency standards, and assessment mechanisms. Under Title I of the ESEA, schools must make adequate yearly progress (AYP) to[ward] ensuring that students who receive Title I services meet these standards. Schools that do not make adequate progress must develop corrective action plans.

In 2001, Congress reauthorized the Elementary and Secondary Education Act and gave the ESEA a new name, The No Child Left Behind Act (NCLB). NCLB greatly expanded the scope of these Title I requirements and reaffirmed the federal government's position that all students should meet high academic standards. In order to obtain funding under Title I, states must develop plans to demonstrate that the state has adopted challenging academic and content standards for all students in the areas of reading or language arts, math and science. These state plans must be developed in coordination with IDEA requirements.

Under NCLB, State content standards must 1) specify what children are expected to know and do; 2) contain rigorous content; and 3) encourage the teaching of advanced skills. State achievement standards must be aligned with content standards and must describe two levels of high achievement: proficient and advanced. These achievement levels determine how well children are mastering the material in the state academic content standards. A third level of achievement called "basic" is required to provide complete information about the progress of students towards meeting the proficient or advanced levels.

NCLB requires that all students, including students with disabilities, be at the proficient or advanced levels by the 2013–2014 school year. All schools must make adequate yearly progress (AYP) towards attaining this goal of all students reaching the proficient or advanced levels. While the specifics of AYP differ from state to state, AYP must be based on student achievement on annual statewide assessment tests that measure the percentage of students who are at the advanced or proficient levels on the state's achievement standards. . . .

Virtually every state has now adopted content and/or proficiency standards that set forth specific performance standards and establish required outcomes for providing students with an adequate or appropriate education under state law. In addition, several states have developed specific assessment measures that test students' levels of achievement in meeting state standards.

Two important aspects of standards based reform relate to FAPE and the U. S. Supreme Court's decision in *Rowley*. First, education standards establish high expectations for all students, including students with disabilities. Such standards assume that all students can achieve high levels of learning if they receive high expectations, clearly defined standards, and effective teaching to support achievement. The intended result of education standards is that all students, including students with disabilities, will learn more. While some states developed specific standards for students with disabilities, most simply created standards that are the same for all students. These high expectations in state education standards are at odds with the core holding in *Rowley* that school districts only need to meet the minimalist "some educational benefit" standard.

The second important aspect of educational standards is the shift from process to outcome. Content and proficiency standards focus on what students actually learn, not the process by which students learn. In general, special education focuses on the process of providing services to students, not on outcomes from these services. Education standards redirect the inquiry to the effectiveness of the education actually provided to students.

This focus on student achievement contradicts the *Rowley* finding that the purpose of the IDEA is to provide access to education, not to address the substance or quality of services students receive once they have access. . . .

Amendments to the IDEA

Congress amended the IDEA in 1997. The 1997 amendments show Congress' intent to incorporate state educational standards into special educational programming for disabled students. The statute now explicitly mandates that states establish performance goals for children with disabilities that are consistent with the goals and standards set for all children. The IDEA now requires states to establish performance indicators to assess their progress toward achieving these goals. At a minimum, goals must include the performance of children with disabilities on assessments, drop out rates, and graduation rates.

The IDEA amendments mark a significant change of direction from the Supreme Court's decision in *Rowley*. These amendments establish high expectations for children with disabilities to achieve real educational results. The amendments change the focus of IDEA from merely providing access to an education, as the Court noted in *Rowley*, to requiring improved results and achievement. These changes were made explicit in the House Committee Report that states:

> This Committee believes that the critical issue now is to place greater emphasis on improving student performance and ensuring that children with disabilities receive a quality public education. Educational achievement for children with disabilities, while improving, is still less than satisfactory.

> This review and authorization of the IDEA is needed to move to the next step of providing special education and related services to children with disabilities: to improve and increase their educational achievement.

Similarly, the findings section of the IDEA now states that:

> Over 20 years of research and experience has demonstrated that the education of children with disabilities can be made more effective by having high expectations for such children

97

and ensuring their access in the general curriculum to the maximum extent possible . . . [and] supporting high-quality, intensive professional development for all personnel who work with such children in order to ensure that they have the skills and knowledge necessary to enable them to meet developmental goals and, to the maximum extent possible, those challenging expectations that have been established for all children.

Whenever possible the general curriculum must now include students with disabilities. Student IEPs must contain goals and objectives that enable disabled students' involvement and progress in the general curriculum. The general curriculum is the curriculum available to all students. Many states base the general curriculum on content and proficiency standards developed by local agencies.

The amended IDEA focuses on the IEP as the primary tool for ensuring that disabled students are included and make progress in the general curriculum. This is one method of incorporating high educational standards into the special education programs of students with disabilities. The IEP details the special education services that must be provided to disabled students. The definition of special education in the IDEA expressly states that special education is specially designed instruction to ensure access to the general curriculum so that the student can meet "the educational standards within the jurisdiction of the public agency that apply to all children." . . .

The 1997 amendments to the IDEA incorporate the high expectations of state educational standards into the programming for disabled students. These amendments demonstrate that FAPE is now more than access to a "basic floor of opportunity." FAPE is now aligned with the high expectations in state education standards. As a result, these high expectations must be incorporated into the IEPs of students with disabilities. . . .

IDEA Goes Well Beyond *Rowley*

The 1997 reauthorization of the IDEA, the emergence of state educational standards as mandated by No Child Left Behind, and constitutional requirements should lead to fundamental changes in how schools write, implement and evaluate Individualized Education Programs (IEPs). This, in turn, should also influence how courts assess FAPE. These changes require a reexamination of *Rowley* and its "some educational benefit" standard.

Reexamining *Rowley* is no small undertaking. *Rowley* has provided the framework for special education services for 20 years. However, the 1997 Amendments to the IDEA make clear that the foundation underlying that reasoning in *Rowley* is no longer present. That is, the IDEA is no longer intended to simply provide students with access to educational services that provide some benefit. The IDEA is intended to go well beyond this by ensuring that students with disabilities receive educational services that incorporate the high expectations in state educational standards and in state court cases regarding an adequate education.

Once these elements are included in the analysis, much of *Rowley* seems inapplicable to questions about the contours of a free and appropriate public education. State educational standards and adequacy requirements now provide the parameters of FAPE. When determining if a school has provided a student with FAPE, courts need to look to these requirements and the extent to which the school provided an Individualized Educational Program that enabled the student to meet these requirements.

> *"My parents only wanted what they thought was best for me, a sign language interpreter to help me fully understand my teacher's spoken words."*

Caught in the Middle of the *Rowley* Litigation

Amy June Rowley

Amy June Rowley, who as a child was at the center of Hendrick Hudson School District v. Rowley, *is an assistant professor at California State University–East Bay, where she coordinates the American Sign Language Program. She recounts in this essay her memories of the events surrounding the 1982 Supreme Court case that changed her family's life so dramatically. In the litigation, Rowley's parents claimed that that the school district ought to provide their daughter, who was deaf, with the appropriate services—a sign-language interpreter—to meet the standards for a free appropriate public education. In a highly personal narrative, Rowley provides background to the case, explaining that when they discovered she was deaf, Rowley's parents decided to send her to the local public school rather than a school for the deaf, in part because the 1975 Education for All Handicapped Children Act (EAHCA) seemed to offer the opportunity for her to receive the kind of education received by hearing children. Tensions with the school district mounted, however, after Rowley's parents requested that their daughter be assigned a sign-language interpreter. Rowley describes her experiences as a deaf child growing up in a school that was often insensitive to her needs. Although many of the teachers and administrators*

Amy June Rowley, "Rowley Revisited: A Personal Narrative," *Journal of Law and Education*, July 1, 2008, pp. 311, 315-28. Reproduced by permission.

had Rowley's interests at heart, she says there was miscommunication and misunderstanding of the needs of a deaf child and an underlying assumption that deaf children are best off communicating with verbal speech. Rowley illustrates how the episode affected her entire family, from her hearing brother being the subject of teasing at school to her parents finally deciding to move away from New York so Amy could attend a school with the support services available to allow her to flourish.

Scholarly legal journals do not usually present this kind of article. Over the years, I have read many articles about *Board of Education of the Hendrick Hudson Central School District v. Rowley*. I have found that almost every article approaches the case from a scholarly perspective. When I have a chance to talk with people about what they have read about the *Rowley* case and what opinions they have formed from those readings, I often find that their perspectives have been significantly influenced by the existing literature. However, almost none of the articles published to date include the personal perspectives of the *Rowley* litigants.

As the child who was at the center of this litigation and who grew up during this case, I want to share my personal experiences. I know not everyone will agree with my perspective. I am not looking for sympathy or support. This is my unique story to share. There are some experiences that I remember vividly—like they happened yesterday. I have emphasized these for the reader in italics. What I hope readers will take away from this article is the understanding that, although educators and litigators often work to help students, some things can happen that are not in the best interest of the students caught in the middle of special education litigation. The same is true for a child caught in the middle of a divorce. Everyone wants to do what is best for the child, but everyone has her own ideas about what is best. This sometimes causes conflicts. In this paper I will show what conflicts arose during the life of the *Rowley* litigation and how I was caught in the middle at times.

After [a] hearing test confirmed that I was deaf, my parents started discussing what educational options were available for me. At the time, it seemed Fanwood The New York School for the Deaf was the only logical choice. I could attend my local elementary school, but, because no one would be signing, I would have no access to the many things that make up the classroom experience, things like specific curriculum content and socialization with the teacher and other students. The local elementary school option was unthinkable to my mom who remembered so clearly the frustration she experienced in school without knowing sign language. It was only after she arrived at Gallaudet [University] and learned sign language that she felt her world had been opened up with full access to information.

Shortly after my parents learned I was deaf, the Education for All Handicapped Children Act, also known as Public Law 94-142, was passed in 1975. This legislation opened the door for disabled children to receive a free and appropriate public education in the least restrictive environment. My parents looked at this new development as an opportunity for me to be mainstreamed and receive an education like that delivered to hearing students. My mom certainly thought this was a better option than the deaf school because, after she learned I was deaf and began to educate me at home, I progressed normally, like hearing children with hearing parents. . . .

Starting School

My mom communicated with Furnace Woods, our local public school, about her desire to have me enroll there. The school administration responded with a willingness to provide necessary services for me, including a sign language interpreter. My brother John was already in school there, and my mom was able to follow up with the school administration about what was needed for my attendance. Furnace Woods had a teletypewriter (TTY) installed. Since my parents had a TTY at home, the school could now call them anytime. Although the staff and administrators at the school seemed to be very sincere about wanting to work with my parents, they were still a part of a larger bureaucratic system, the Hendrick Hudson School District, and were required to report to the Superintendent. Any action at the school level, such as providing a sign language interpreter, would have to be approved by the district office.

When I started kindergarten, my parents expected that an interpreter would be present in my class. When one was not there, my parents asked why one had not been provided. These inquiries created tension between the school district and my parents. My parents only wanted what they thought was best for me, a sign language interpreter to help me fully understand my teacher's spoken words. Hendrick Hudson School District was advised by its lawyer to exhaust all other options first. My mother was not willing to put my education on hold while everyone could agree on exactly what I needed. She talked with my teachers every day and made sure at home that I learned what was taught at school. Thus, in every sense of the word, I was home schooled even though I was also attending Furnace Woods School.

Eventually an agreement was reached that placed an interpreter in the classroom on a "trial basis" for four weeks.

One day this man shows up in my class. I know he is the interpreter because my mom has told me he will be coming. But I am scared. I don't know what an interpreter is. I have never seen one before. I am only five, and I don't know what I am supposed to do with him. He also looks scary. He is very tall to anyone who is little like me, and he is wearing standard interpreter attire of all black clothes. But I don't know that white interpreters wear dark colors to contrast with their skin color.

No one in kindergarten is wearing all black so there must be something wrong with him. I am even more scared. I am only so eager to walk away and keep myself occupied with other doings. Once in a while I quickly steal a glance at him and see him signing. I wonder why. I did not understand that he was signing what the teacher was saying.

To further complicate things, there were several observers in class, and I knew somehow that they were there because of the man in black. I could not wait until the entourage and the oddly dressed, tall man would leave so my kindergarten class could get back to normal. Due to my reaction, the interpreter was removed from my classroom after only two weeks. The tension between my parents and the school district was heating up.

I can feel it, but not from my parents. I feel it at school.

Wishing for Things to Be Normal

I progressed into first grade and had a new teacher, who was very different from my kindergarten teacher. She didn't teach me or make sure I was following everything. Since I was already a good reader, I recall always working on worksheets that required I answer questions about books I had read. I cannot remember ever doing anything else in her classroom, but I am sure I did. What I do remember is that there was a steady stream of visitors, and I could clearly see that my teacher was displeased with the interruptions caused by the visitors. It was almost as if she had lost all control of her classroom. And who bore the brunt of her frustration? Me.

During that year, I also had a teacher of the deaf, Sue Williams. She would pull me out of class to make sure I was able to follow along. When I could not follow along in my normal class, she would teach me what I did not understand. I greatly resisted these meetings because it drew more attention to me and made me look like I was totally responsible for all the disruptions going on in class. In his book, *A Case about Amy*, R.C. Smith was able to use excerpts from Sue Williams's diary to document my frustration. The entry for February 16, 1979 shows the dialogue that took place between Sue Williams and me:

Feb 16. Had a heart-to-heart with Amy, who acted as if she didn't want to come with me. I asked her how she was feeling.

"I feel bad," Amy said. "I don't want to come with you."

"What's wrong?"

"I don't know"

"Amy, what did you think of the man who visited yesterday?"

"I don't like those things."

"What do you mean by 'things'?"

"All of the people coming."

"How does your mother feel?"

"She thinks I need an interpreter because I don't understand anything."

"Amy, you seem to understand things, not everything, but most things."

"Yes."

"Do you understand Mrs. Globerman?"

"Yes, everything she says."

"Well, what don't you understand?"

"I don't understand library."

"You mean the stories? You don't understand them?"

"Yes."

"You want to understand what's happening right?"

"Right."

"What about movies?"

"I don't understand them much."

I remember so well how I always insisted I understood everything at the time. This was a defense mechanism I used so everyone would leave me alone and things would just return to normal. This was an interesting goal for me. At this point of my life I had never really been exposed to "a normal classroom environment." I am not sure why I resisted everything so much. I suspect I was able to pick up on body language and emotions better than I was able to pick up spoken words, and the emotions made a big impact on me when I could see others felt uncomfortable. One thing I do know is that I preferred to be with the other students all the time rather than being constantly removed from class to meet with my deaf education teacher, going to speech class, or leaving for testing. Sue Williams recognized these feelings and tried to work with me in my class rather than taking me out. This arrangement was ideal for me, but it was bothersome for the classroom teacher. I was no longer paying attention to her. I was working with Sue Williams instead. In addition, other parents were complaining to my teacher because Sue Williams was using sign language in the classroom with me. I seemed to be the only one who wanted to stay in the classroom. No one else wanted me to stay.

Second Grade

When I moved into second grade, many of the frustrations that I had been experiencing did not subside. I reacted by continuing to resist and act out.

During second grade tensions are at their highest. I am very aware of things happening all around me. Before, the principal, Joseph Zavarella, would come to my class occasionally. Now he comes to my class every day. My parents have already won one hearing at the federal level and an appeal is under way. Every year my parents have an Individualized Education Plan (IEP) meeting with the school, and every year my parents refuse to sign it because there is nothing on it related to provision of interpreting services. The rest of the stuff on the IEP is the school's defense that they are trying to provide me with the best possible service they think I need (without an interpreter, of course).

The controversial IEP included providing speech classes to improve my ability to make others understand me, but this did not help *me* understand *others*. Wasn't that the point? I was required to wear an FM system with the teacher wearing a microphone. The FM system certainly amplified everything, but I heard only sounds. I could understand nothing. Simple amplification of the sounds did not allow comprehension of the meaning of the sounds. I think it is sometimes difficult for hearing people to understand that hearing aids and FM systems do not have the same effect as eyeglasses. I imagine the noises I heard everyday sounded like loud power tools to hearing people. This constantly bugged me, and I was happy to turn the noises off. I recall many times that the noises in my head certainly were a distraction as I watched the teacher. I remember reading that the school contended that I had a lot of residual hearing so they felt it was their obligation to make sure I was able to use it. That comment was a light bulb moment for me. It showed me how much hearing people really don't understand what deaf people actually hear. Every deaf person has a different audiogram, and every deaf person reacts differently to their environment. If two deaf people with a similar audiogram were compared based on their audiograms only, one would find a lot of similarities. However, if one looks at both people to see how they function and how they communicate, the audiogram is often not an accurate representation of who deaf people are.

Third Grade

With second grade out of the way, I was on to a new start in third grade. The overall environment improved for me because the school and my parents seemed to have stopped fighting. There were fewer disruptions to my class, and we settled into everyday routines easily. In the lawsuit, the school district lost at the district court level and again at the Court of Appeals. After they lost the appeal, the school district was required to provide me with an interpreter. Having an interpreter in class could have been considered a "new distraction," but the interpreter quickly inserted herself into our everyday routine. Soon many of my classmates and I could not imagine our class without her. For the first time, I really enjoyed school. I was able to follow along perfectly in classroom discussions, and my interpreter made sure to interpret everything, including my classmates' conversations.

My interpreter, Fran Miller, had deaf parents so she grew up communicating in sign language. Not only was she fluent in signing, she was also a skilled interpreter and fully understood how to be a language mediator. She did just that, mediating exchanges among the other students, the teacher and me. I felt friendships blossoming, and I could communicate and follow group conversations. Because I was fluent in sign language, the interpreter opened up a new avenue of complete accessibility for me. I enjoyed school now. I looked forward to recess. The interpreter would follow me out and help me and other children figure out what we wanted to do. Before Fran Miller became my interpreter I had always followed the other children outside. They usually wanted to play kickball, but I was often not included. I would go to the playground and play alone or with a few other children. Now, when other children were in a group discussing what they wanted to do, I could be a part of the group. My interpreter also interpreted those conversations. I finally felt I had a voice because I could say I wanted to play kickball, and they would make sure I was involved. An added bonus of having an interpreter in the classroom meant that, when I got home from school, I only had to do my homework. I no longer had to work with my mother when I got home to relearn everything I was supposed to have learned in class that day. Now I really had a lot more time to play and "just be a kid." Third grade was a really good year.

Resentment Toward My Family

School seemed really good, and life "seemed back to normal," but things were actively brewing in the background. When R.C. Smith was researching the experiences of everyone involved with the proceedings, he was able to find the notes of people who came to visit the school and witnessed the escalation of such hostilities. Mary Sheie was the lead expert witness that my parents' lawyer used, and she made several visits to Furnace Woods. In a note Mary Sheie commented on "how surprised she was at how much anger there was in the classroom and in the principal's office and how calmly [my mom] had taken it." This was written in reference to a visit by other expert witnesses my parents used in the trial. Why was it okay to have the school's witnesses in the classroom but not my parents' witnesses? During that same visit Mary Sheie went to the principal's office with my mother and noted that the principal practically scolded my mother, saying the school had provided so many things like the TTY and the FM system and never once had my mother said thanks. There was so much anger because the school was taking steps to accommodate me, but those steps never included the one thing my parents requested—an interpreter.

My brother had to transfer to a private school about twenty minutes away because it became too difficult for him to continue to go to Furnace Woods Elementary. Many of his classmates and their parents did not understand what was going on between my parents and the school district, and there was much hostility directed at my brother. As the only hearing person in my immediate family, he was able to hear and understand the comments from people around him. I am sure that my parents and I had people making comments around us, but we were not as aware of it as my brother was. When John transferred to a new school, he found that his problems followed him there. Students made fun of him and picked on him because his family was different; we were all odd. *Who else had a deaf family? Probably no one else.* Deaf families are a rarity, and a family with one hearing child and other deaf children is even more unusual. Most deaf people have several hearing children, and those hearing siblings are able to support each other. John had no one. Even as siblings, we were worlds apart. We were fighting the same battle but fighting it separately. It was almost like we were not struggling against the same thing, making our struggles seem more lonely and more difficult.

When my situation at school had improved, my parents finally had the time to address my brother's situation, but much damage had already been done. The resentment that the school district and the community had towards my family was there and likely to remain forever. People who had direct interaction with my parents or me were very supportive, but others who did not know us and only saw us on TV or read about us in newspapers often felt strongly that we had no place in the public schools.

Early in the legal proceedings, the school made it clear that I should have attended Fanwood so they would not have to be responsible for the costs of supportive services. However, as the case progressed, their position changed. They were no longer were able to prove Fanwood was a good fit for me and agreed with my parents that Furnace Woods was where I belonged. What services I should receive to be successfully integrated at Furnace Woods continued to be debated. I underwent many observations and was tested by various psychologists. The school hired their own psychologist for several different kinds of tests, including IQ tests. Their psychologist did not sign so my parents challenged the validity of the results. They got their own signing psychologist who could fully communicate with me. The results of the tests were different, and it was later admitted into evidence that I was very smart, a high functioning child with a lot of potential. The school district could no longer claim that I would be better off at Fanwood. I was on grade level and would be ahead of many deaf peers who had not learned anything until they entered school. . . .

The Case

In March 1982, while I was in fourth grade, the United States Supreme Court heard the oral argument in the case between Hendrick Hudson School District and my parents. My parents' lawyer, Michael Chatoff, was the first deaf person ever to argue before the Supreme Court. Michael became deaf during law school due to tumors on his auditory nerves. Surgery to remove the tumors cut his auditory nerves, and he became permanently deaf. He struggled with neurofibromatosis [a condition that causes tumors to grows on nerve tissue], but it did not keep him from becoming a lawyer. Through chance, he met my parents and decided to take on our case. He never charged my parents any legal fees, which would have been huge by the time the case finally came to an end. Since he became deaf as an adult, he preferred to talk instead of signing. English was his first language. The Supreme Court arranged for the court proceedings to be transferred to a computer by a transcriptionist so Michael could read everything that was going on in real time. This was the first time such a venture had been undertaken. It is now common practice in courts all over America.

During the summer between fourth grade and fifth grade, the Supreme Court announced that the two previous decisions of the lower courts in my parents' favor were overturned. The Supreme Court sided with the school district, finding that the school did provide me with adequate services to make sure I was passing from grade to grade. For the Court, a free and appropriate public education did not mean I was entitled to reach my full potential as the gifted child that I was. It just meant that as long as I was passing, I was doing fine.

My parents had already decided to move to New Jersey. There was no reason to stay in Peekskill, New York. I would never have an interpreter in school there. My father commuted between New York and New Jersey every day for many years so it seemed logical to move closer to where my father worked. In New Jersey, there was a day school for the deaf where many deaf children were mainstreamed. However, before we could move, I had to stick out one more year at Furnace Woods. . . .

A New School, a New Life

When my parents put their house up for sale, the school district found out that we were moving and put a lien on our house to recover their costs in the litigation. We moved anyway, but my parents were not able to sell their house. The lien did not make matters easier. The conflict between the school district and my parents continued and became a dogfight. Living in New York was bad for my family, and it was quickly getting worse.

The move to New Jersey was the best thing that happened to my family. I started attending school with other deaf kids. For the first time I truly didn't feel alone. I had an interpreter in all my classes. My brother had many friends who didn't care that his parents and his sister were deaf. They saw deaf students every day so the idea of deaf families was not such a foreign concept for them. Finally, I was no longer abnormal just because I was deaf.

I remember more than I would like to remember about my experience at Furnace Woods. I believe that I am supposed to remember so I can share my story in the hope that other children do not have to experience the same things I did. My experience informs the kind of decisions I make today as an adult. If a conflict arises and I know that I will have to put someone in an uncomfortable situation, I am more likely to avoid it. However, conflict and discomfort can't always be avoided. I wish both sides had not had to go into litigation. I wish that we had not had to move to find a new school district so that my needs could be met.

Children should be allowed to be children. Too often children are robbed of their right to grow up without the weight of the world on their shoulders. I know the weight of my world was squashing me in elementary school as my family and I pursued the educational experience I needed and deserved. Many times I wanted to play or be like the little kid I should have been, but I was expected to be just the opposite. With the case going all the way to the Supreme Court, I got a lot of national attention from the media. I didn't ask for that. People ask me if this was all worth it. Would I do this again? I was faced with that decision with my own children who are deaf. The school district I first worked with informed me that they wanted my oldest daughter to be able to function without an interpreter by the time she entered school. In my mind I was thinking that the school wanted to make her hearing. They wanted to deprive me and her of communication. I had to explain to the school that American Sign Language is not a detriment to my daughter's education but actually an advantage that helps her thrive in school. Twenty-five years ago my parents asked for an interpreter for the exact same reasons.

Twenty-five years later I know there has been progress, but it is not always evident. So would I do it again? Not at the expense of my children.

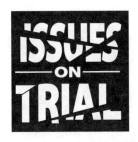

CHAPTER 3

Affirming the Rights of Disabled People to Participate in Community Life

Case Overview

Olmstead v. L.C. and E.W. (1999)

Lois Curtis and Elaine Wilson (L.C. and E.W.), two women with mental disabilities, had been voluntarily committed to Georgia Regional Hospital at Atlanta (GRH). After a time, the women indicated their preference for discharge; their treatment professionals also recommended release into community programs. The state, however, refused their request. The Atlanta Legal Aid Society filed a lawsuit in 1995 on their behalf, claiming violation of rights guaranteed under the Americans with Disabilities Act (ADA).

The ADA is a plenary civil rights statute designed to stop practices that segregate persons with disabilities. Title II of the ADA prohibits a public entity from excluding any persons, by reason of their disability, from its services, programs, or activities. To implement Title II, the Department of Justice adopted an "integration regulation" requiring public agencies to "administer services, programs, and activities in the most integrated setting appropriate to the needs of qualified individuals with disabilities." But agencies were only required to make "reasonable modifications" to avoid discrimination and need not "fundamentally alter" the nature of their programs. The case hinged on the meaning and scope of the integration regulation: Was a community-based treatment facility the most integrated setting appropriate for Curtis and Wilson? Would the provision of community-based treatment require Georgia to fundamentally alter its programs?

The state of Georgia argued that lack of funds, not discrimination, was the reason for the plaintiffs' continued institutionalization. In addition, it maintained that it could not immediately transfer them without fundamentally altering its programs. The lower courts rejected both of these defenses. In its ruling, the Eleventh Circuit Court set a high bar for a judgment of "fundamental alteration," and for the inclusion of cost as a factor influencing the choice of treatment facilities. (The district court had deemed Georgia's cost defense irrelevant.)

In 1999 Justice Ruth Bader Ginsburg, writing for the majority, denied Georgia's petition, concluding that Title II requires states to place people with disabilities "in community settings rather than institutions when (a) treatment professionals recommend community placement, (b) the affected individual consents, and (c) the state can reasonably accommodate the placement, taking into account resource limits and the needs of others with mental disabilities. Ginsburg also argued, more generally, that segregation becomes discriminatory when institutionalization perpetuates "unwarranted assumptions that persons so isolated are incapable or unworthy of participating in community life" and when institutional life "severely diminishes individuals' everyday life activities." In such situations, discrimination exists because such persons are required, because they are disabled, to pay a much higher social price to receive treatment than their nondisabled counterparts. Thus, services to persons with mental disabilities should take place "in the most integrated setting possible."

Justice Clarence Thomas's dissent focused on the majority's nonstandard interpretation of the term "discrimination." The majority, he claimed, adopted a broader definition than Congress intended when it enacted the ADA and, moreover, the definition deviated from that used by the Court in a string of prior discrimination cases. "At bottom," Thomas concluded, "the type of claim approved of by the majority does not concern a prohibition against certain conduct (the traditional understanding of discrimination), but rather imposition of a standard of care. . . . By adopting such a broad view of discrimination, the majority drains the term of any meaning other than as a proxy for decisions disapproved of by this Court."

Olmstead v. L.C. challenges public agencies to increase the range of community-based care options available to persons with mental disabilities. *Olmstead*, however, made only limited recommendations to states about what constitutes a "reasonable accommodation" to their care systems. To determine when the requirements are met, lower courts have looked for effort and progress in adding community-based services.

> *"The State's responsibility, once it pro-*
> *vides community-based treatment to*
> *qualified persons with disabilities, is*
> *not boundless."*

Majority Opinion: States Must Make Reasonable Efforts to Provide Community-Based Services for the Disabled

Ruth Bader Ginsburg

Ruth Bader Ginsburg was appointed to the Supreme Court by President Bill Clinton in 1993. In her written opinion in the case of Olmstead v. L.C. and E.W., *she affirms a ruling by the United States Court of Appeals for the Eleventh Circuit that unnecessary segregation of individuals with disabilities is discrimination based on disability. In 1995 the Atlanta Legal Aid Society filed a case against the state of Georgia on behalf of Lois Curtis and Elaine Wilson, alleging that the two plaintiffs were being isolated in a psychiatric institution when, with proper supports, they could enjoy a more normal life in a community setting. The Eleventh Circuit Court of Appeals ruled in 1997 that the state's failure to provide integrated community services under these circumstances did indeed violate the Americans with Disabilities Act (ADA). The state of Georgia appealed to the Supreme Court to decide whether the public services portion of the ADA "compels the state to provide treatment and habilitation for mentally disabled persons in a community placement, when appropriate treatment and habilitation can also be provided to them in a*

Ruth Bader Ginsburg, majority opinion, *Olmstead v. L.C. and E.W.*, U.S. Supreme Court, 1999.

State mental institution." In her written opinion, Ginsburg answers the question with a qualified "yes." She writes that unjustified institutionalization is discriminatory because it perpetuates stereotypes, suggests that people with disabilities are undeserving of participating in community life, and curtails everyday life activities such as family relations, work, and cultural enrichment. People with disabilities cannot be forced to choose between receiving appropriate medical services and relinquishing their basic civil rights. However, the state's obligation is not absolute and must be balanced with considerations of its resources, costs of providing community-based care, the range of services it provides others with mental disabilities, and its obligations to provide services equitably.

This case concerns the proper construction of the antidiscrimination provision contained in the public services portion of the Americans with Disabilities Act (ADA) of 1990. Specifically, we confront the question whether the proscription of discrimination may require placement of persons with mental disabilities in community settings rather than in institutions. The answer, we hold, is a qualified yes. Such action is in order when the State's treatment professionals have determined that community placement is appropriate, the transfer from institutional care to a less restrictive setting is not opposed by the affected individual, and the placement can be reasonably accommodated, taking into account the resources available to the State and the needs of others with mental disabilities. . . .

This case, as it comes to us, presents no constitutional question. The complaints filed by plaintiffs-respondents L. C. and E. W. did include such an issue; L. C. and E. W. alleged that defendants-petitioners, Georgia health care officials, failed to afford them minimally adequate care and freedom from undue restraint, in violation of their rights under the Due Process Clause of the Fourteenth Amendment.

Discrimination Continues to Be a Problem

In the opening provisions of the ADA, Congress stated findings applicable to the statute in all its parts. Most relevant to this case, Congress determined that

> "(2) historically, society has tended to isolate and segregate individuals with disabilities, and, despite some improvements, such forms of discrimination against individuals with disabilities continue to be a serious and pervasive social problem;
>
> "(3) discrimination against individuals with disabilities persists in such critical areas as . . . institutionalization . . .;
>
> . . .
>
> "(5) individuals with disabilities continually encounter various forms of discrimination, including outright intentional exclusion, . . . failure to make modifications to existing facilities and practices, . . . [and] segregation. . . ."

Congress then set forth prohibitions against discrimination in employment, public services furnished by governmental entities, and public accommodations provided by private entities. The statute as a whole is intended "to provide a clear and comprehensive national mandate for the elimination of discrimination against individuals with disabilities." . . .

Facts of the Case

Respondents L. C. and E. W. are mentally retarded women; L. C. has also been diagnosed with schizophrenia, and E. W., with a personality disorder. Both women have a history of treatment in institutional settings. In May 1992, L. C. was voluntarily admitted to Georgia Regional Hospital at Atlanta (GRH), where she was confined for treatment in a psychiatric unit. By May 1993, her psychiatric condition had stabilized, and L. C.'s treatment team at GRH agreed that her needs could be met appropriately in one of the community-based programs the State supported. Despite this evaluation, L. C. remained institutionalized until February 1996, when the State placed her in a community-based treatment program.

E. W. was voluntarily admitted to GRH in February 1995; like L. C., E. W. was confined for treatment in a psychiatric unit. In March 1995, GRH sought to discharge E. W. to a homeless shelter, but abandoned that plan after her attorney filed an administrative complaint. By 1996, E. W.'s treating psychiatrist concluded that she could be treated appropriately in a community-based setting. She nonetheless remained institutionalized until a few months after the District Court issued its judgment in this case in 1997.

In May 1995, when she was still institutionalized at GRH, L. C. filed suit in the United States District Court for the Northern District of Georgia, challenging her continued confinement in a segregated environment. Her complaint invoked 42 U. S. C. §1983 and provisions of the ADA, §§12131–12134, and named as defendants, now petitioners, the Commissioner of the Georgia Department of Human Resources, the Superintendent of GRH, and the Executive Director of the Fulton County Regional Board (collectively, the State). L. C. alleged that the State's failure to place her in a community-based program, once her treating professionals determined that such placement was appropriate, violated, *inter alia* [among other things], Title II of the ADA. L. C.'s pleading requested, among other things, that the State place her in a community care residential program, and that she receive treatment with the ultimate goal of integrating her into the mainstream of society. E. W. intervened in the action, stating an identical claim.

Lower Courts' Findings

The District Court granted partial summary judgment in favor of L. C. and E. W. The court held that the State's failure to place L. C. and E. W. in an appropriate community-based treatment program violated Title II of the ADA. In so ruling, the court rejected the State's argument that inadequate funding, not discrimination against L. C. and E. W. "by reason of" their disabilities, accounted for their retention at GRH. Under Title II, the court concluded, "unnecessary institutional segregation of the disabled constitutes discrimination *per se*, which cannot be justified by a lack of funding."

In addition to contending that L. C. and E. W. had not shown discrimination "by reason of [their] disabilit[ies]," the State resisted court intervention on the ground that requiring immediate transfers in cases of this order would "fundamentally alter" the State's activity. The State reasserted that it was already using all available funds to provide services to other persons with disabilities. Rejecting the State's "fundamental alteration" defense, the court observed that existing state programs provided community-based treatment of the kind for which L. C. and E. W. qualified, and that the State could "provide services to plaintiffs in the community at considerably *less* cost than is required to maintain them in an institution."

The Court of Appeals for the Eleventh Circuit affirmed the judgment of the District Court, but remanded for reassessment of the State's cost-based defense. As the appeals court read the statute and regulations: When "a disabled individual's treating professionals find that a community-based placement is appropriate for that individual, the ADA imposes a duty to provide treatment in a community setting—the most integrated setting appropriate to that patient's needs"; "[w]here there is no such finding [by the treating professionals], nothing in the ADA requires the deinstitutionalization of th[e] patient."

The Court of Appeals recognized that the State's duty to provide integrated services "is not absolute"; under the Attorney General's Title II regulation, "reasonable modifications" were required of the State, but fundamental alterations were not demanded. The appeals court thought it clear, however, that "Congress wanted to permit a cost defense only in the most limited of circumstances." In conclusion, the court stated that a cost justification would fail "[u]nless the State can prove that requiring it to [expend additional funds in order to provide L. C. and E. W. with integrated services] would be so unreasonable given the demands of the State's mental health budget that it would fundamentally alter the service [the State] provides." Because it appeared that the District Court had entirely ruled out a "lack of funding" justification, the appeals court remanded, repeating that the District Court should consider, among other things, "whether the additional expenditures necessary to treat L. C. and E. W. in community-based care would be unreasonable given the demands of the State's mental health budget." ...

Attorney General's Findings

Endeavoring to carry out Congress' instruction to issue regulations implementing Title II, the Attorney General, in the integration and reasonable-modifications regulations, made two key determinations. The first concerned the scope of the ADA's discrimination proscription, the second concerned the obligation of the States to counter discrimination. As to the first, the Attorney General concluded that unjustified placement or retention of persons in institutions, severely limiting their exposure to the outside community, constitutes a form of discrimination based on disability prohibited by Title II. ("A public entity shall administer services ... in the most integrated setting appropriate to the needs of qualified individuals with disabilities.") Regarding the States' obligation to avoid unjustified isolation of individuals with disabilities, the Attorney General provided that States could resist modifications that "would fundamentally alter the nature of the service, program, or activity."

The Court of Appeals essentially upheld the Attorney General's construction of the ADA. As just recounted, the appeals court ruled that the unjustified institutionalization of persons with mental disabilities violated Title II; the court then remanded with instructions to measure the cost of caring for L. C. and E. W. in a community-based facility against the State's mental health budget. . . .

The Question of Discrimination

We examine first whether, as the Eleventh Circuit held, undue institutionalization qualifies as discrimination "by reason of . . . disability." The Department of Justice has consistently advocated that it does. Because the Department is the agency directed by Congress to issue regulations implementing Title II, its views warrant respect. . . .

The State argues that L. C. and E. W. encountered no discrimination "by reason of" their disabilities because they were not denied community placement on account of those disabilities. Nor were they subjected to "discrimination," the State contends, because "'discrimination' necessarily requires uneven treatment of similarly situated individuals," and L. C. and E. W. had identified no comparison class, *i.e.*, no similarly situated individuals given preferential treatment. We are satisfied that Congress had a more comprehensive view of the concept of discrimination advanced in the ADA.

The ADA stepped up earlier measures to secure opportunities for people with developmental disabilities to enjoy the benefits of community living. The Developmentally Disabled Assistance and Bill of Rights Act (DDABRA), a 1975 measure, stated in aspirational terms that "[t]he treatment, services, and habilitation for a person with developmental disabilities . . . *should be* provided in the setting that is least restrictive of the person's personal liberty." . . . Ultimately, in the ADA, enacted in 1990, Congress not only required all public entities to refrain from discrimination; additionally, in findings applicable to the entire statute, Congress explicitly identified unjustified "segregation" of persons with disabilities as a "for[m] of discrimination."

Recognition that unjustified institutional isolation of persons with disabilities is a form of discrimination reflects two evident judgments. First, institutional placement of persons who can handle and benefit from community settings perpetuates unwarranted assumptions that persons so isolated are incapable or unworthy of participating in community life. Second, confinement in an institution severely diminishes the everyday life activities of individuals, including family relations, social contacts, work options, economic independence, educational advancement, and cultural enrichment. . . .

We emphasize that nothing in the ADA or its implementing regulations condones termination of institutional settings for persons unable to handle or benefit from community settings. Title II provides only that "qualified individual[s] with a disability" may not "be subjected to discrimination."

Consistent with these provisions, the State generally may rely on the reasonable assessments of its own professionals in determining whether an individual "meets the essential eligibility requirements" for habilitation in a community-based program. Absent such qualification, it would be inappropriate to remove a patient from the more restrictive setting.

Limits on the State's Responsibilities

The State's responsibility, once it provides community-based treatment to qualified persons with disabilities, is not boundless. The reasonable-modifications regulation speaks of "reasonable modifications" to avoid discrimination, and allows States to resist modifications that entail a "fundamenta[l] alter[ation]" of the States' services and programs. The Court of Appeals construed this regulation to permit a cost-based defense "only in the most limited of circumstances," and remanded to the District Court to consider, among other things, "whether the additional expenditures necessary to treat L. C. and E. W. in community-based care would be unreasonable given the demands of the State's mental health budget."

The Court of Appeals' construction of the reasonable-modifications regulation is unacceptable for it would leave the State virtually defenseless once it is shown that the plaintiff is qualified for the service or program she seeks. If the expense entailed in placing one or two people in a community-based treatment program is properly measured for reasonableness against the State's entire mental health budget, it is unlikely that a State, relying on the fundamental-alteration defense, could ever prevail. . . .

To maintain a range of facilities and to administer services with an even hand, the State must have more leeway than the courts below understood the fundamental-alteration defense to allow. If, for example, the State were to demonstrate that it had a comprehensive, effectively working plan for placing qualified persons with mental disabilities in less restrictive settings, and a waiting list that moved at a reasonable pace not controlled by the State's endeavors to keep its institutions fully populated, the reasonable-modifications standard would be met. . . . In such circumstances, a court would have no warrant effectively to order displacement of persons at the top of the community-based treatment waiting list by individuals lower down who commenced civil actions.

For the reasons stated, we conclude that, under Title II of the ADA, States are required to provide community-based treatment for persons with mental disabilities when the State's treatment professionals determine that such placement is appropriate, the affected persons do not oppose such treatment, and the placement can be reasonably accommodated, taking into account the resources available to the State and the needs of others with mental disabilities. The judgment of the Eleventh Circuit is therefore affirmed in part and vacated in part, and the case is remanded for further proceedings consistent with this opinion.

"Temporary exclusion from community
placement does not amount to 'discrimination.'"

Dissenting Opinion: *Olmstead* Did Not Involve Discrimination

Clarence Thomas

Clarence Thomas has served as an associate justice of the U.S. Supreme Court since 1991. He was appointed by President George H.W. Bush. In a dissenting opinion in Olmstead v. L.C. and E.W., *Thomas argues that the majority's interpretation of discrimination in the ruling was not in line with judicial history. The Court had decided in* Olmstead *that "unjustified institutional isolation" is a form of discrimination that constitutes an abridgement of a person's basic civil rights. The state of Georgia, it held, was discriminating when it continued to segregate Lois Curtis and Elaine Wilson in a mental institution when they wanted to move out and when professional psychiatrists had agreed that they were ready for community-based living. Thomas argues that the majority ruling is unsatisfactory for a number of reasons. Temporary exclusion from community placement, he insists, is not the same as discrimination. He notes that the Court has never endorsed an interpretation of the term* discrimination *encompassing disparate treatment among members of the same protected class. He maintains that the case at hand is about a standard of care and not about prohibition against certain conduct, which is the traditional understanding of dis-*

Clarence Thomas, dissenting opinion, *Olmstead v. L.C. and E.W.*, U.S. Supreme Court, 1999.

crimination. *Thomas expresses concern that the majority opinion imposes significant federalism costs, directing states on how to make decisions about the delivery of public services and forcing them to defend themselves in federal court every time resources prevent the immediate placement of a qualified individual.*

Title II of the Americans with Disabilities Act of 1990 (ADA), provides:

> "Subject to the provisions of this subchapter, no qualified individual with a disability shall, *by reason of such disability*, be excluded from participation in or be denied the benefits of the services, programs, or activities of a public entity, *or be subjected to discrimination* by any such entity" (emphasis added).

The majority concludes that petitioners "discriminated" against respondents—as a matter of law—by continuing to treat them in an institutional setting after they became eligible for community placement. I disagree. Temporary exclusion from community placement does not amount to "discrimination" in the traditional sense of the word, nor have respondents shown that petitioners "discriminated" against them "by reason of" their disabilities.

The Nature of Discrimination

Until today, this Court has never endorsed an interpretation of the term "discrimination" that encompassed disparate treatment among members of the *same* protected class. Discrimination, as typically understood, requires a showing that a claimant received differential treatment vis-à-vis members of a different group on the basis of a statutorily described characteristic. This interpretation comports with dictionary definitions of the term "discrimination," which means to "distinguish," to "differentiate," or to make a "distinction in favor of or against, a person or thing based on the group, class, or category to which that person or thing belongs rather than on individual merit."

Our decisions construing various statutory prohibitions against "discrimination" have not wavered from this path. The best place to begin is with Title VII of the Civil Rights Act of 1964, as amended, the paradigmatic anti-discrimination law: Title VII makes it "an unlawful employment practice for an employer . . . to *discriminate* against any individual with respect to his compensation, terms, conditions, or privileges of employment, because of such individual's race, color, religion, sex, or national origin" (emphasis added). We have explained that this language is designed "to achieve equality of employment opportunities and remove barriers that have operated in the past to favor an identifiable group of white employees over other employees."

Under Title VII, a finding of discrimination requires a comparison of otherwise similarly situated persons who are in different groups by reason of certain characteristics provided by statute. For this reason, we have described as "nonsensical" the comparison of the racial composition of different classes of job categories in determining whether there existed disparate impact discrimination with respect to a particular job category. . . .

A "Capacious" Understanding of "Discrimination"

Despite [the] traditional understanding, the majority derives a more "capacious" [capable of containing a great deal] definition of "discrimination," as that term is used in Title II of the ADA, one that includes "institutional isolation of persons with disabilities." It chiefly relies on certain congressional findings contained within the ADA. To be sure, those findings appear to equate institutional isolation with segregation, and thereby discrimination. The congressional findings, however, are written in general, hortatory [encouraging] terms and provide little guidance to the interpretation of the specific language. . . . In my view, the vague congressional findings upon which the majority relies simply do not suffice to show that Congress sought to overturn a well-established understanding of a statutory term (here, "discrimination"). Moreover, the majority fails to explain why terms in the findings should be given a medical content, pertaining to the place where a mentally retarded person is treated. When read in context, the findings instead suggest that terms such as "segregation" were used in a more general sense, pertaining to matters such as access to employment, facilities, and transportation. Absent a clear directive to the contrary, we must read "discrimination" in light of the common understanding of the term. We cannot expand the meaning of the term "discrimination" in order to invalidate policies we may find unfortunate. . . .

Addressing Standard of Care

At bottom, the type of claim approved of by the majority does not concern a prohibition against certain conduct (the traditional understanding of "discrimination"), but rather imposition of a standard of care. As such, the majority can offer no principle limiting this new species of "discrimination" claim apart from an affirmative defense because it looks merely to an individual in isolation, without comparing him to otherwise similarly situated persons, and determines that discrimination occurs merely because that individual does not receive the treatment he wishes to receive. By adopting such a broad view of discrimination, the majority drains the term of any meaning other than as a proxy for decisions disapproved of by this Court.

Costs to Federalism

Further, I fear that the majority's approach imposes significant federalism costs, directing States how to make decisions about their delivery of public services. We previously have recognized that constitutional principles of federalism erect limits on the Federal Government's ability to direct state officers or to interfere with the functions of state governments. . . .

Disability Not Cause of Exclusion

Finally, it is also clear petitioners did not "discriminate" against respondents "by reason of [their] disabili[ties]," as §12132 [of the ADA] requires. We have previously interpreted the phrase "by reason of" as requiring proximate causation. Such an interpretation is in keeping with the vernacular understanding of the phrase. This statute should be read as requiring proximate causation as well. Respondents do not contend that their disabilities constituted the proximate cause for their exclusion. Nor could they—community placement simply is not available to those without disabilities. Continued institutional treatment of persons who, though now deemed treatable in a community placement, must wait their turn for placement, does not establish that the denial of community placement occurred "by reason of" their disability. Rather, it establishes no more than the fact that petitioners have limited resources.

"One of the major barriers to enhancing the supply of home and community-based care has been the institutional bias of Medicaid."

Olmstead Raised More Issues than It Resolved

Randy Desonia

Randy Desonia was a senior research associate at the National Health Policy Forum when he wrote the following viewpoint. His viewpoint lays the groundwork for understanding the implications of the ruling in Olmstead v. L.C. and E.W., *which he says has far-reaching consequences for the long-term care of people with disabilities. The case was brought in Georgia by Atlanta Legal Aid on behalf of Lois Curtis and Elaine Wilson, who lived in a state psychiatric hospital. After several years of treatment, doctors and caretakers agreed that they were qualified for placement in the community. Georgia had allocated few resources to community placements, but had focused on funding large institutions and nursing facilities. Thus, even though the women wanted to live in a community placement, they were forced to continue to live in an institution. They filed suit in federal court in Atlanta to enforce their rights under the Americans with Disabilities Act (ADA). They won their case, and the state was required to place them in the community. The state appealed, but the federal appeals court agreed that the ADA required that the women be served in the community. The Supreme Court affirmed the federal appeals court's decision. Desonia says that while the decision at first set off a flurry of activity, it has in fact*

Randy Desonia, "Is Community Care a Right? The Unfolding Saga of the *Olmstead* Decision," *NHPF Background Paper*, March 12, 2003. Reproduced by permission.

resulted in a great deal of uncertainty. Desonia reviews the critical components influencing the case, including Medicaid's role in funding community-based care. He states that one of the most difficult issues is that Medicaid, the primary payer of long-term care services, has historically favored institutional care over community-based services. Desonia goes on to describe the federal and state responses to the ruling and discusses some of the legal issues surrounding the decision that still need to be addressed.

On June 19, 1999, the U.S. Supreme Court handed down a landmark civil rights decision that caused people with disabilities to cheer. The ruling, *Olmstead v. L.C.*, put states on notice that unnecessary segregation of individuals with disabilities is a violation of the Americans with Disabilities Act of 1990 (ADA). People with disabilities hailed the ruling as their civil rights equivalent to *Brown v. Board of Education of Topeka*, which ordered the desegregation of the nation's public schools. A new era promising home- and community-based services as the standard for long-term care was on the horizon.

The ruling elicited powerful responses from many organizations and people. The federal government issued new guidance for states to comply with the ADA and provided grants to expand the availability of community-based services. Dozens of states organized task forces to develop implementation plans. Researchers published numerous legal analyses. And advocates filed lawsuits against states.

Although the case that set off this flurry of activity appears straight-forward, the decision it produced has resulted in years of uncertainty. The Court's opinion is complex, its guidance to states is vague, and the unanswered legal questions are many. Writing for the majority, Justice Ruth Bader Ginsburg foreshadowed the uncertainties the opinion would leave behind when she wrote: "We confront the question whether the proscription of discrimination may require placement of persons with mental disabilities in community settings, rather than in institutions. The answer, we hold, is a qualified yes." Resolving the ambiguities raised by this ruling will take many more years. In the meantime, states have no choice but to proceed with their efforts to comply.

The *Olmstead* case is not based on Medicaid law, nor does it expressly require a restructuring of the program. However, the *Olmstead* plaintiffs sought placement under a Medicaid home- and community-based services waiver, and state compliance with the ADA will likely be financed largely by Medicaid. Consequently, the first step in understanding the *Olmstead* ruling is a brief review of Medicaid's evolving role in financing home- and community-based care.

Medicaid's Institutional Bias

Medicaid is the nation's primary payer of long-term care services, paying 44 percent of such costs in 2000. Twenty-seven percent of that amount pays for services delivered in home- and community-based settings. This represents a four-fold increase in such Medicaid expenditures since 1990. Despite this growth, however, there remains substantial unmet demand, and waiting lists for services are common.

One of the major barriers to enhancing the supply of home and community-based care has been the institutional bias of Medicaid; that is, its historic inclination to cover long-term care services more readily when the beneficiary resides in an institution, such as a nursing home, than when he or she lives at home. When Medicaid was created in the 1960s, the home health care industry was not very developed, and Medicaid's service coverage for long-term care was focused on nursing homes. The only mandatory coverage of long-term care services was for skilled nursing facility care for people age 21 and older, although states had the option of providing some home health services, private-duty services, and rehabilitation services.

There were a few additions to home-based services during the 1970s, such as mandatory coverage of home health services for those entitled to skilled nursing facility services. However, a broad range of home- and community-based services were not added. Policymakers feared runaway costs would result from induced demand, also referred to as the "woodwork effect." Consequently, the vast majority of Medicaid long-term care spending continued to be for nursing home care.

In the late 1970s and early 1980s, a series of demonstrations were conducted to measure whether providing community-based services to a Medicaid beneficiary was less expensive than institutional care. These studies helped generate policymaker interest in using home- and community-based services as a substitute for nursing home care, even before many of these demonstrations were evaluated. In 1981, Congress amended Section 1915 of the Social Security Act, authorizing states, subject to federal approval, to cover home- and community-based services under a waiver program.

Under the Section 1915(c) waiver authority, states could provide home- and community-based services to specific Medicaid populations such as the aged disabled and people with mental retardation or developmental disabilities. The law listed several types of services allowed under a waiver (for example, homemaker, home health aide, and adult day health) but also permitted other services, as long as they were cost-effective and necessary to avoid institutionalization.

The growth of Medicaid home- and community-based care, however, was restrained by waiver policies and procedures to protect against the woodwork effect. First, the population eligible for a waiver was restricted by requiring that the person not only needed the care but also, after an assessment, was determined to be at risk for placement in an institution. Second, the maximum number of people that could be placed in a waiver was capped based on a formula (frequently referred to as the "cold bed rule") that measured bed vacancies in nursing homes. Third, in response to great concern over costs at the federal level, especially within the Office of Management and Budget, the size of the waiver programs and the pace of approvals were restrained.

The major breakthrough came in 1993 when President [Bill] Clinton announced to the nation's governors that the Centers for Medicare and Medicaid Services (CMS, then named the Health Care Financing Administration) would provide greater waiver flexibility for states. The next year CMS eliminated the cold bed rule. In its place, CMS substituted a more flexible cost-neutrality requirement, under which states had to demonstrate that aggregate expenditures with the waiver program would not exceed the cost of serving an equivalent group of people in an institution.

The result was a dramatic increase in state spending for home- and community-based services. In 1990, Medicaid spent $3.9 billion on home and community-based care, representing 13 percent of total Medicaid long-term care spending. By 2000, the amount had increased more than four-fold, to $18.2 billion, or 27 percent of total Medicaid spending for long-term care. In 1999, 49 states had 212 waivers serving a total of 688,152 people.

Despite these improvements, a number of factors still discourage the growth in Medicaid home- and community-based care. One is a payment policy that does not cover housing or meal costs in the home-based setting, although Medicaid does factor these costs into payments to nursing homes. This distinction furthers the contention that an institutional bias against home- and community-based care still exists.

Another factor is states' concern over their budget outlays. With Medicaid second only to education as the largest state expenditure, states have moved to control home- and community-based service costs by restricting (by age and conditions) the populations eligible for the services, the number of slots for each waiver, the service cost per person, and the covered services. In addition, states may be cautious in filling all approved slots, preferring to wait until they are confident that sufficient monies are available for the state match.

The cumulative effect of these factors has been numerous waiting lists for waiver programs. For example, one report noted that in the mid-1990s New Hampshire had a waiting list of 325 people; New Mexico, 2,400; Massachusetts, 2,437; Florida, 6,000; and Texas, 17,500. The lists can be so long that some people wait years before receiving services. This shortage of a full array of readily available home- and community-based services created the environment for the *Olmstead* decision.

State Responses

State reaction to the *Olmstead* ruling was also swift and broad in scope. By the end of 2000, 37 states had task forces or work groups to develop comprehensive plans or significant papers that could serve as blueprints of change. The size and representativeness of these work groups was extensive. The few states that did not initiate specific *Olmstead* planning activities argued they were already implementing efforts to improve the availability of community-based services. For example, Vermont has no institution for people with developmental disabilities, and all nursing home residents have been assessed for community-based services. Oregon has a six-year plan to eliminate a waiting list of 5,000 individuals desiring services under a home- and community-based waiver. Nonetheless, these two states were among the 48 that received systems change grants.

A review of the state plans and papers issued either in final or draft form found several common, long-standing barriers to complying with the *Olmstead* ruling—barriers that are difficult and often expensive to surmount. Compounding these obstacles is the current state fiscal crisis. Recent shortfalls have constrained the growth in resources available for financing expansions in Medicaid services, including home- and community-based services, and have likely diverted the attention of Medicaid long-term care staff toward the immediate need to contain Medicaid costs. In light of such difficult barriers and a tight fiscal environment, implementation of *Olmstead* might be expected to grind to a halt in virtually all states.

In fact, while states' progress in complying with the *Olmstead* decision may have slowed somewhat compared to the initial burst of activity, planning and design activity continues. One reason for this continued activity has been the systems change grants. The combination of grant funds and the existence of a technical collaborative has enabled fiscally stressed states to maintain some staff time devoted to *Olmstead* and have the access to a national network of expert assistance necessary to design and implement.

Another force behind continued state activity has been the pressure created by the legal challenges filed by people with disabilities. These cases constitute the next stage in *Olmstead* implementation. They will be instrumental in deciding how many people will be protected by the ADA and in which settings (for example, only institutional or also the community). They will also determine how quickly people with disabilities will receive home-care services.

Implementation: District Court Rulings

Care must be taken when examining the many *Olmstead*-related court cases, for very few have completed the trial phase, much less been subjected to review by the appellate courts. While it is tempting to select cases that may serve as precedents, such an effort is fraught with peril. Each case has unique circumstances that may mitigate its likelihood of serving as a precedent. Successfully picking the "right one" is unlikely. This predicament is exacerbated by the relative dearth of precise guidance from the regulations issued under Title II of the ADA and the absence of case law regarding fundamental alteration within the context of community-based care. It will take years for the key issues to wend their way through the courts before case law is built and precedents handed down.

Nonetheless, looking at the *Olmstead* decision and a few key rulings by the district courts does reveal some of the emerging policy issues courts will struggle with in the coming years:

- Will the courts interpret broadly who is covered by the *Olmstead* ruling?

- Will courts require home placements when waiver slots are available, as in the original *Olmstead* case?

- After existing waiver slots are filled, will the courts require states to expand their waiver programs, resulting in sustained long-term expansion of home care services?

The courts' rulings on the range of individuals covered by *Olmstead* will have a major impact on both people with disabilities and state and federal budgets. Since the *Olmstead* plaintiffs had developmental disabilities and were residing in a state psychiatric hospital, the Supreme Court's majority opinion considered its decision within the context of mental disabilities, state mental health budgets, and state psychiatric institutions. The ADA, however, covers people with all types of disabilities—physical as well as mental; it also covers people living in other types of institutions, such as nursing homes, and those living in the community.

Numbers Affected by *Olmstead*

Currently, there is no reliable estimate for the number of people who may benefit from the ruling. There are approximately 34 million people with severe disabilities and 10.4 million people with disabilities so severe that they need some level of personal assistance. The General Accounting Office (GAO), which has a more conservative approach to the disability numbers, estimates that there are 2.3 million adults with severe disabilities living in the community who need considerable assistance from another person. And, it estimates, there are approximately 1.8 million people with disabilities that are living in institutions (that is, nursing facilities, institutions for the mentally retarded and developmentally disabled, and state or county facilities for the mentally ill).

The GAO did not relate these figures to the number of people to whom *Olmstead* may apply. It concluded that there was too much uncertainty about the widely varying population of people with disabilities, the settings in which they are receiving services, and their true risk of institutionalization to make such an estimate. Thus, one must look elsewhere to provide some illumination of who may potentially benefit from the ruling.

The conditions of people with disabilities seeking remedies in the courts are similar to those of the *Olmstead* plaintiffs. The most extensive and frequently updated listing of *Olmstead*-related lawsuits is by Human Services Research Institute (HSRI). In 10 states, the plaintiffs have a developmental disability or are mentally retarded, are residing in institutions, and are seeking community placements. If this trend is to continue, the reach of *Olmstead* will still be important but limited in scope.

However, there is the potential for greater pressure in broadening the scope of *Olmstead*. Four other cases have at least some plaintiffs who have physical disabilities. The most recent is a Georgia case filed on January 31, 2003; in *Birdsong et al. v. Perdue*, a class action complaint has been filed on behalf of individuals with physical disabilities who reside in nursing homes or are at risk of nursing home placement. The suit alleges that Georgia has made no significant effort to expand home- and community-based services since the *Olmstead* decision.

Another study by the Center for Health Services Research and Policy at the George Washington University supports the argument that pressure is building for a broader scope of *Olmstead*. The study examined the characteristics of people who have filed a Title II ADA-related complaint with the DHHS [Department of Health and Human Services] Office of Civil Rights (OCR) and found that many differed from those of the plaintiffs in *Olmstead* and *Olmstead*-related lawsuits. For example, 50 percent of those who filed an OCR complaint were people with physical disabilities. In terms of living arrangements, 42 percent were in nursing homes, and 30 percent were residing in the community (most of them living with families).

One substantial subgroup of people with disabilities does not constitute a significant proportion in either study—people with disabilities who are age 65 and older. This is surprising because aging advocates played an active role in many of the state *Olmstead* workgroups. However, no conclusions can be drawn from the HSRI and OCR studies since their methodologies may underestimate the true involvement of the aged in *Olmstead*-related efforts. If the aged disabled increase their participation in future legal cases, *Olmstead* could have a larger impact.

Another Critical Issue

A second critical issue courts will grapple with is whether to require the states to place people in existing home- and community-based services waiver programs. In the *Olmstead* case, Georgia had vacant slots under a waiver program that fit the needs of the plaintiffs. The waiver slots were vacant because the state had not allocated state funding. A question the district courts are facing, but few have decided, is whether fulfilling a request for a placement is a reasonable modification when slots are available.

In post-*Olmstead* settlement agreements, many states are filling vacant slots and expanding their home- and community-based services waiver programs to include more slots. Over a five-year period, Massachusetts will extend community services to an additional 375 to 400 people per year. Hawaii has agreed to increase the number of waiver slots by 70 percent over a three-year period. Louisiana, Washington, and West Virginia have also signed agreements to expand the number of waiver slots.

Not all states, however, are filling vacant slots. In response to the state fiscal crisis, Michigan and Idaho proposed reducing the number of filled waiver slots. Michigan's proposal is being challenged in court. In one district case, *Benjamin v. Ohl*, the federal district court instructed the state that it "will have to show more than that the state has not appropriated enough funding."

Expansion Potential

A third critical question that courts will need to address in determining whether states' efforts meet the reasonable-modifications standard involves what to do when a state's waiver slots are filled: Will courts require states to obtain new waivers or will they be allowed to have their waiting lists grow? One interpretation is that instructing the state to expand its waiver program would constitute a "fundamental alteration," since it might require the state to reallocate budget funds from a disability program to finance a waiver expansion. This could violate Ginsburg's admonition that states "mete out services with an even hand."

It is not clear how the courts will rule on this issue. As noted, in response to *Olmstead*-related lawsuits, several states have signed settlement agreements expanding the number of waiver slots. But those settlements were signed between February 2000 and August 2001, when state budgets were in good shape. No similarly broad agreements have been crafted since then [as of early 2003].

One case, *Arc of Washington State v. Lyle Quasim*, did touch on this issue. The federal district judge made a summary ruling dismissing the case. The dismissal was based on the finding that the ADA cannot serve as the basis for ordering a state to increase its limit on the number of individuals who receive waiver services. Doing so would require the state to make a "fundamental alteration" in its services. This case, however, eventually resulted in a settlement agreement signed in April 2001.

If other courts hand down decisions that adopt the argument of the judge in *Arc of Washington v. Lyle Quasim*, a deterrent for expanding the supply of home- and community-based services could be created. States, knowing that obtaining more waiver slots will place them under great legal pressure to fill them immediately, may decide not to request additional slots.

If this disincentive were to occur, *Olmstead* could slow the expansion of new waiver slots—the exact opposite of what advocates are seeking. The overall effect of *Olmstead* could simply be a short-term spurt in funding unfilled home- and community-based service waiver slots, followed by slow growth thereafter. However, adopting the scenario in Ginsburg's two-part example—an effective plan and a waiting list moving at a reasonable pace—could lead to a quite different conclusion.

For a state to demonstrate it has met the first criterion in the example—a "comprehensive, effectively working plan for placing qualified persons with mental disabilities in less restrictive settings"—implies that it must be making continued progress in improving the availability of community placements. The district courts will have to rule on what constitutes such a plan. Although there is no systematic report on the implementation status of state plans, one study of plans in 14 states found that their implementation would put those states in compliance with the *Olmstead* decision. In only one case (*Arc of Delaware v. Meconi*), which has yet to go to trial, has the plaintiff argued that the state's plan is inadequate.

Determining whether a state is conforming to the second part of the Court's example—"a waiting list that moved at a reasonable pace"—is more problematic: A state may have a difficult time arguing it is complying with Title II of the ADA if the waiting list for waiver slots remains static or moves very slowly. While no decisions based on the ADA have focused exclusively on what constitutes a reasonable pace, a set of court cases focused on Medicaid waiting lists could provide precedents for defining it.

Under Medicaid law, services are to be provided with "reasonable promptness." In a watershed decision, the 11th Circuit Court of Appeals ruled federal Medicaid law does not allow a state to wait-list individuals for ICF/MR (intermediate care facilities for the mentally retarded) waiver services indefinitely. While reasonable promptness has not been precisely defined, there appears to be a growing consensus among some courts that frequent waiting periods of "many years are outside of the zone of reasonableness." Thus, in the longer term, the Ginsburg example may provide people with disabilities additional support in challenging states that hope to be in compliance simply by filling vacant waiver slots without ever expanding their waiver programs. . . .

Unanswered Questions

Care must be taken in estimating the power of *Olmstead* to effect change. Regardless of future court decisions, there are still many issues impeding the expansion of home- and community-based long-term services that are not addressed by *Olmstead*. It does not increase the workforce needed to deliver more services, nor does it create an oversight system assuring that the community-based services delivered are of high quality. A number of questions are yet to be answered if home- and community-based care are to be expanded:

- How can the true extent of the "woodwork effect" on the demand for services in the community setting be determined?

- Will the federal government provide states additional assistance in meeting their obligations?

- Will the New Freedom Initiative [a 2001 federal action to improve access to community living for the disabled], including the systems change grants, be able to meet the high expectations for removing barriers to community care at the federal and state levels?

- Are there other state financing strategies that can be developed to fund an increase in services?

Although *Olmstead* is not the solution to bridging the large gap between demand and supply for home- and community-based services, it does apply additional pressure on state and federal policymakers to address these issues. And it adds another stakeholder in the process—judges who will be determining whether the pace of implementation is adequate.

How powerful this force will be is yet to be determined. Nonetheless, the ruling has served as a catalyst for state and federal government activity. It has empowered people with disabilities, particularly those residing in institutions, with legal recourse to obtain home- and community-based services. And the Court's opinion has set into motion a new expectation for community-based services that will be hard to ignore. Long-term care policymakers will find it difficult not to make some accommodation to this ruling today and in the years to come.

"Not surprisingly, the Court's ruling [in Olmstead] did not end the policy debate. And now, . . . the controversy is heating up again."

Olmstead Did Not End Debate over Institutional vs. Communal Living for the Disabled

Michael Levin-Epstein

Michael Levin-Epstein is editor in chief of the Food and Drug Law Institute. In the following essay, he comments on how three lawsuits, filed in 2005 and 2006, have reopened the controversy surrounding community-based care for people with disabilities. He explains that the even though in 1999 the Supreme Court ruled in Olmstead v. L.C. and E.W. *that under the Americans with Disabilities Act that states can be required to place individuals with mental disabilities in community settings rather than institutions, many people are not being moved to more integrated care settings. Levin-Epstein reviews the details of the cases and presents the views of people on both side of the debate about the feasibility of providing community-based care when it is desired. Even those who support integrated care for some people point out that lack of resources is an issue, as is the lack of community acceptance of people with mental illness. Others note that nursing home care is a complex issue, as there are some people with disabilities who never get better, some who need care for only part of the day, and some patients whom the state does not want to keep in mental institutions as they get older and have other needs. Because community-care providers do not always take the initiative, oftentimes institutionalized settings are the best available option. As one professional working in the field of providing care for the aging points out, even if nursing homes are not the ideal place for some people, they do receive good care in those facilities. This is a point that continues to be debated, however.*

For decades, healthcare policy wonks have debated whether adults with mental illnesses should be housed in nursing homes. Then, in 1999, the Supreme Court ruled in *Olmstead v. L. C. and E. W.* that under the Americans with Disabilities Act (ADA), states can be required to place individuals with mental disabilities in community settings rather than institutions.

The key issues in placement, according to the Court, are:

- Do treatment professionals think that community placement is appropriate for an individual?

- Does the individual oppose transfer to a less restrictive setting?

- Can placement be reasonably accommodated, taking into account a state's resources and the needs of others with mental disabilities?

Not surprisingly, the Court's ruling did not end the policy debate. And now, as the result of three lawsuits filed in federal courts, the controversy is heating up again.

Three New Lawsuits

In the first lawsuit, filed in August 2005, the American Civil Liberties Union of Illinois, along with the Bazelon Center for Mental Health Law, the organization Equip for Equality, and the law firm Kirkland and Ellis, alleged that four mentally ill residents of nursing homes were being needlessly segregated and inappropriately "warehoused" in violation of federal law. The ACLU is seeking class-action status for the plaintiffs against nursing homes that are institutions for mental diseases (IMDs), according to lead attorney Benjamin Wolf.

"Many, if not all, of the persons at these facilities could be served in more integrated settings in the community," Wolf asserts. "However, as a country we have been slow to make those accommodations for individuals with mental illnesses."

In February 2006, another lawsuit accused the state of Connecticut of forcing psychiatric patients into nursing homes when community living would provide more suitable alternatives. Connecticut Lt. Gov. Kevin Sullivan is championing efforts to make sure that individuals with mental illnesses are placed in community-based care rather than nursing homes. Nursing home beds are far more costly than home or community care, Sullivan notes. The situation that prompted the lawsuit is "wrong as a matter of law and as a matter of smart public policy," he says. "Nursing homes do not provide effective care and recovery for the nongeriatric mental health patients who are trapped there." And it shouldn't take a lawsuit to make Connecticut do the "right thing," Sullivan adds.

The third suit was filed in March 2006, claiming that New York State officials violated the ADA by transferring mentally ill patients from state psychiatric hospitals into locked nursing home units.

Need for Appropriate Placement

Each lawsuit has different details, but they all involve seeking more appropriate placement for individuals with mental illnesses, says Jennifer Mathis, the Bazelon Center's deputy legal director. "Nursing homes are not designed to serve that population. They're set up to serve people with more intensive healthcare needs," she says. For the most part, Mathis explains, people with mental illnesses do not fall into that category.

"These are not people who are walking around with IVs [intravenous medication apparatuses]," she notes. Mathis asserts that these individuals generally are capable of being in the community and living normal lives, but instead they are being institutionalized, sometimes in locked nursing home units. "It appears that states are moving backwards rather than forward in warehousing people," she concludes.

"Inconsistent data" make it impossible to determine accurately the number of mentally ill individuals states are housing in nursing homes, according to a recent report from the Department of Health and Human Services's Office of the Inspector General [OIG], but as many as 20% of residents in such facilities might have some form of mental disorder. What is clear is that many states are not doing enough to identify, screen, or treat younger adults (ages 22 to 64) with mental illnesses in nursing facilities, the OIG reports. Access to mental health services within nursing facilities also appears to be a problem, with as many as half of nursing homes unable to provide adequate psychiatric consultation.

It adds up to a tragic situation, says Linda Rosenberg, president and CEO of the National Council for Community Behavioral Healthcare. "To be sent to a nursing home is especially sad when it's avoidable," Rosenberg says. "Nursing home care is very expensive, and if even a portion of those funds were directed to rent and individualized support, people with mental illness currently in nursing homes could live in the community." Rosenberg adds that "States must be pressed into taking advantage of increasing Medicaid flexibility, and create community-based services as alternatives to inappropriate and unnecessary use of nursing homes."

The federal government (through the Deficit Reduction Act) recently offered states such flexibility. The Centers for Medicare and Medicaid Services' "Money Follows the Person" program invites states to apply for federal matching funds to implement initiatives that move people out of institutional settings, such as nursing homes, and into the community.

Complex Issues

Inappropriate placement of mentally ill patients should be avoided whenever possible, agrees nursing home CEO Melvin Siegel, chairman of the legislative committee of the Illinois Nursing Home Administrators Association. However, economic issues, the limited availability of facilities, and the lack of community acceptance of people with mental illnesses often leave no choice but to place such individuals in nursing homes, he explains.

In addition, Siegel says many nursing home residents could not function in smaller community-based settings without a significant increase in staffing. "They need a degree of assistance and supervision that's not feasible in community facilities without a significant increase in costs," he says. Without such assistance and supervision, some mentally ill individuals would not be able to perform daily living activities, take their medications as needed, or eat properly. The latter is a particular problem for those with diabetes and a mental illness, notes Siegel.

Siegel adds that most individuals with mental illness placed in nursing homes are not there for life. "They're there until they learn the skills they need," he says.

Nursing home placement is a vexing, complicated issue, agrees Gary Moak, MD, president of the American Association for Geriatric Psychiatry. First, there's overlapping responsibility between the long-term care industry and state mental health departments. In addition, he says, many elderly people in nursing homes, who need nursing home care, have late-life mental disorders, and there also are people with chronic mental health conditions whom states don't want to keep in state hospitals as they get older, he explains.

Many people with illnesses such as bipolar disorder, major depression, and schizophrenia never get 100% better and cannot manage basic life skills, notes Dr. Moak. "They may need to be supervised through parts of the day. Where should they be best cared for?" he asks.

Before the 1970s, such persons would have lived in state mental hospitals, Dr. Moak recalls. But all that changed with the deinstitutionalization movement. Recent revisions to federal nursing home regulation, such as Preadmission Screening and Resident Review (PASRR) requirements, specifically are aimed at keeping persons with mental disorders out of nursing homes unless state authorities find that those persons need 24-hour medical care.

Lack of Community-Based Providers

Yet community-based providers have not always stepped up to the plate to fill the void, according to Dr. Moak. "A nursing home is not the best option for some patients. But it may be the only option," he says.

Indeed, says Mary Giliberti, director of public policy and advocacy at the National Alliance on Mental Illness, the lack of community-based services often results in persons with mental illnesses winding up in jails, prisons, or nursing homes. "We're concerned about transinstitutionalization,'" which goes counter to placing persons with mental illness in the least restrictive environment, she asserts.

In some cases, people with a treatable disability who are admitted into a nursing home might function better and be able to meet the demands of a less restrictive setting if they received better therapy, including newer drugs, concludes Dr. Moak.

But even if individuals with mental illnesses end up in nursing homes, it doesn't mean they are not being cared for properly, says Margaret Morelli, president of the Connecticut Association of Not-for-Profit Providers for the Aging. "Nursing home placement may not be ideal for some persons with mental illness," she explains, but "they all receive good care." That's a point, however, likely to be debated by advocates on the other side, as the question of where people with mental illnesses can best function is again taken to the courts.

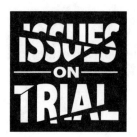

CHAPTER 4

Ensuring Equal Access to Public Places

Case Overview

Tennessee v. Lane and Jones (2004)

George Lane and Beverly Jones, both paraplegics, lacked access to state and county courthouses because the buildings were not wheelchair accessible. As a result, Jones, a court reporter, lost work, and Lane, a defendant, was required to crawl or be carried up two flights of stairs to attend his own trial. This, they argued, was a violation of their rights granted in Title II of the Americans with Disabilities Act (ADA), which states that "public entities" may not deny disabled persons access to their "services, programs, or activities." In 1998 Lane and Jones brought suit against the state of Tennessee.

Tennessee challenged the appropriateness of this law, claiming Eleventh Amendment sovereign immunity. The Eleventh Amendment, ratified in 1795, protects state sovereignty by stipulating they cannot be sued by private parties in federal courts. In some cases, however, Congress can override states' sovereign immunity. Section five of the Fourteenth Amendment grants Congress power to enact "appropriate" legislation to enforce the amendment's provisions. *Tennessee v. Lane and Jones* represents yet another stage in the Court's interpretation of section five of the Fourteenth Amendment.

Since Title II of the ADA was enacted as a means of enforcing the Due Process Clause of the Fourteenth Amendment, the questions before the Court concerned the appropriateness of this legislation. Did Congress overstep its bounds when it enacted the law? Was Title II a valid exercise of Congress's power to enforce the Fourteenth Amendment's prohibition of discrimination?

To judge the appropriateness of Title II, Justice John Paul Stevens, writing for the majority, used a test developed in an earlier case, *City of Boerne v. Flores* (1997). That case found that remedies and preventive measures designed to address discrimination cannot create a "substantive change in governing law." Legislation must exhibit "a congruence and proportionality between the injury to be prevented or remedied and the means adopted to that end." The question, then, was whether Title II passed *Boerne*'s "congruence and proportionality" test.

Application of this test required two broad judgments. First, the Court had to agree that the constitutional violations at stake were serious. It did. Stevens noted that Title II was a response to a history of pervasive and systematic rights violations by public agencies against people with disabilities. In this case, several violations were identified. Among the most important was the denial of a "meaningful opportunity to be heard" in court.

Second, the Court had to focus not just on the seriousness of the problem but on the cost of the solution. Tennessee had argued that these costs could be unreasonably high. Stevens pointed out that the Court was only required to address one of Title II's many applications, and thus the act's breadth was not a problem. He then noted that states are required to take only reasonable measures to provide accessibility. In no case must a state be forced to "undertake measures that would impose an undue financial or administrative burden." Therefore, Title II was a valid exercise of Congress's authority to enforce Fourteenth Amendment guarantees.

In his dissent, Justice William Rehnquist argued that the majority's decision was inconsistent with *Alabama v. Garrett* (2001), that Congress did not intend Title II to be used as a means for remedying violations of due process, and that inaccessible public buildings do not violate any right to due process.

The merits and impact of *Lane* continue to be debated. There is still uncertainty about the intended goals of the ADA, the extent to which it provides an exception to Eleventh

Amendment sovereign immunity, and about whether things such as carpal tunnel syndrome, breast cancer, or a bad back deserve the same protections and accommodations as blindness, deafness, or paraplegia.

> "Ordinary considerations of cost and convenience alone cannot justify a State's failure to provide individuals with a meaningful right of access to the courts."

Majority Opinion: States Must Take Reasonable Steps to Accommodate People with Disabilities

John Paul Stevens

John Paul Stevens, the senior associate justice of the U.S. Supreme Court, was appointed to the bench by Gerald Ford in 1975. In his written opinion in the case of Tennessee v. Lane and Jones, *Stevens maintains that Title II of the Americans with Disabilities Act (ADA) did not violate the sovereign immunity doctrine of the Eleventh Amendment when it allowed individuals to sue states for denying them services based on their disabilities. The case began when George Lane and Beverly Jones, both with mobility impairments, sued the state of Tennessee for failing to ensure that courthouses were accessible to people with disabilities. Jones, a court reporter, and Lane, a defendant in a criminal case, had been denied access to courtrooms on the second floors of buildings that had no elevators. Tennessee moved to dismiss the suit on grounds of "sovereign immunity" (the Eleventh Amendment's prohibition of lawsuits against states in federal courts). The U.S. district court denied the state's motion, and Tennessee appealed to the U.S. Court of Appeals for the*

John Paul Stevens, majority opinion, *Tennessee v. Lane and Jones*, U.S. Supreme Court, 2004.

Sixth Circuit, which affirmed the trial court's decision. In a five-to-four decision, the Supreme Court upheld the lower courts' rulings. Stevens writes that Congress had sufficiently demonstrated that people with disabilities had been denied the right to exercise fundamental rights protected by the Due Process Clause of the Fourteenth Amendment, such as access to a court. This "pattern of unequal treatment" violates the Constitution, and victims of such discrimination may sue the state, he contends. Furthermore, Stevens states that the remedies required by Congress are not unreasonable but congruent and proportional—and therefore constitutional—because the "reasonable accommodations" mandated by the ADA to allow people with disabilities to exercise their rights were not unduly burdensome and disproportionate to the harm.

Title II of the Americans with Disabilities Act of 1990 (ADA or Act), provides that "no qualified individual with a disability shall, by reason of such disability, be excluded from participation in or be denied the benefits of the services, programs or activities of a public entity, or be subjected to discrimination by any such entity." The question presented in this case is whether Title II exceeds Congress' power under §5 of the Fourteenth Amendment.

In August 1998, respondents George Lane and Beverly Jones filed this action against the State of Tennessee and a number of Tennessee counties, alleging past and ongoing violations of Title II. Respondents, both of whom are paraplegics who use wheelchairs for mobility, claimed that they were denied access to, and the services of, the state court system by reason of their disabilities. Lane alleged that he was compelled to appear to answer a set of criminal charges on the second floor of a county courthouse that had no elevator. At his first appearance, Lane crawled up two flights of stairs to get to the courtroom. When Lane returned to the courthouse for a hearing, he refused to crawl again or to be carried by officers to the courtroom; he consequently was arrested and jailed for failure to appear. Jones, a certified court reporter, alleged that she has not been able to gain access to a number of county courthouses, and, as a result, has lost both work and an opportunity to participate in the judicial process. Respondents sought damages and equitable relief.

The State moved to dismiss the suit on the ground that it was barred by the Eleventh Amendment. The District Court denied the motion without opinion, and the State appealed. The United States intervened to defend Title II's abrogation [violation] of the States' Eleventh Amendment immunity. On April 28, 2000, after the appeal had been briefed and argued, the Court of Appeals for the Sixth Circuit entered an order holding the case in abeyance [temporary inactivity] pending our decision in *Board of Trustees of Univ. of Ala. v. Garrett....*

The ADA, Congress, and Discrimination

The ADA was passed by large majorities in both Houses of Congress after decades of deliberation and investigation into the need for comprehensive legislation to address discrimination against persons with disabilities. In the years immediately preceding the ADA's enactment, Congress held 13 hearings and created a special task force that gathered evidence from every State in the Union. The conclusions Congress drew from this evidence are set forth in the task force and Committee Reports, described in lengthy legislative hearings, and summarized in the preamble to the statute. Central among these conclusions was Congress' finding that

> individuals with disabilities are a discrete and insular minority who have been faced with restrictions and limitations, subjected to a history of purposeful unequal treatment, and relegated to a position of political powerlessness in our society, based on characteristics that are beyond the control of such individuals and resulting from stereotypic assumptions not truly indicative of the individual ability of such individuals to participate in, and contribute to, society.

Invoking "the sweep of congressional authority, including the power to enforce the fourteenth amendment and to regulate commerce," the ADA is designed "to provide a clear and comprehensive national mandate for the elimination of discrimination against individuals with disabilities." It forbids discrimination against persons with disabilities in three major areas of public life: employment, which is covered by Title I of the statute; public services, programs, and activities, which are the subject of Title II; and public accommodations, which are covered by Title III.

Title II prohibits any public entity from discriminating against "qualified" persons with disabilities in the provision or operation of public services, programs, or activities. The Act defines the term "public entity" to include state and local governments, as well as their agencies and instrumentalities. Persons with disabilities are "qualified" if they, "with or without reasonable modifications to rules, policies, or practices, the removal of architectural, communication, or transportation barriers, or the provision of auxiliary aids and services, meet the essential eligibility requirements for the receipt of services or the participation in programs or activities provided by a public entity." Title II's enforcement provision incorporates by reference §505 of the Rehabilitation Act of 1973, which authorizes private citizens to bring suits for money damages. . . .

Congress Meant to Abrogate States' Immunity

The Eleventh Amendment renders the States immune from "any suit in law or equity, commenced or prosecuted . . . by Citizens of another State, or by Citizens or Subjects of any Foreign State." Even though the Amendment "by its terms . . . applies only to suits against a State by citizens of another State," our cases have repeatedly held that this immunity also applies to unconsented suits brought by a State's own citizens. Our cases have also held that Congress may abrogate the

State's Eleventh Amendment immunity. To determine whether it has done so in any given case, we "must resolve two predicate questions: first, whether Congress unequivocally expressed its intent to abrogate that immunity; and second, if it did, whether Congress acted pursuant to a valid grant of constitutional authority."

The first question is easily answered in this case. The Act specifically provides: "A State shall not be immune under the eleventh amendment to the Constitution of the United States from an action in Federal or State court of competent jurisdiction for a violation of this chapter." As in [*Alabama v.*] *Garrett*, no party disputes the adequacy of that expression of Congress' intent to abrogate the States' Eleventh Amendment immunity. The question, then, is whether Congress had the power to give effect to its intent. . . .

Rights Enforced in Title II

The first step [to determine whether Congress had the power to abrogate the State's Eleventh Amendment Immunity] . . . requires us to identify the constitutional right or rights that Congress sought to enforce when it enacted Title II. In *Garrett* we identified Title I's purpose as enforcement of the Fourteenth Amendment's command that "all persons similarly situated should be treated alike." As we observed, classifications based on disability violate that constitutional command if they lack a rational relationship to a legitimate governmental purpose.

Title II, like Title I, seeks to enforce this prohibition on irrational disability discrimination. But it also seeks to enforce a variety of other basic constitutional guarantees, infringements of which are subject to more searching judicial review. These rights include some, like the right of access to the courts at issue in this case, that are protected by the Due Process Clause of the Fourteenth Amendment. The Due Process Clause and the Confrontation Clause of the Sixth Amendment, as applied to the States via the Fourteenth Amendment, both guarantee to a criminal defendant such as respondent Lane the "right to be present at all stages of the trial where his absence might frustrate the fairness of the proceedings." The Due Process Clause also requires the States to afford certain civil litigants a "meaningful opportunity to be heard" by removing obstacles to their full participation in judicial proceedings. We have held that the Sixth Amendment guarantees to criminal defendants the right to trial by a jury composed of a fair cross section of the community, noting that the exclusion of "identifiable segments playing major roles in the community cannot be squared with the constitutional concept of jury trial." And, finally, we have recognized that members of the public have a right of access to criminal proceedings secured by the First Amendment.

Whether Title II validly enforces these constitutional rights is a question that "must be judged with reference to the historical experience which it reflects." While §5 authorizes Congress to enact reasonably prophylactic remedial legislation, the appropriateness of the remedy depends on the gravity of the harm it seeks to prevent. "Difficult and intractable problems often require powerful remedies," but it is also true that "[s]trong measures appropriate to address one harm may be an unwarranted response to another, lesser one." . . .

With respect to the particular services at issue in this case, Congress learned that many individuals, in many States across the country, were being excluded from courthouses and court proceedings by reason of their disabilities. A report before Congress showed that some 76% of public services and programs housed in state-owned buildings were inaccessible to and unusable by persons with disabilities, even taking into account the possibility that the services and programs might be restructured or relocated to other parts of the buildings. Congress itself heard testimony from persons with disabilities who described the physical inaccessibility of local courthouses. And its appointed task force heard numerous examples of the exclusion of persons with disabilities from state judicial services and programs, including exclusion of persons with visual impairments and hearing impairments from jury service, failure of state and local governments to provide interpretive services for the hearing impaired, failure to permit the testimony of adults with developmental disabilities in abuse cases, and failure to make courtrooms accessible to witnesses with physical disabilities. . . .

The conclusion that Congress drew from this body of evidence is set forth in the text of the ADA itself: "[D]iscrimination against individuals with disabilities persists in such critical areas as . . . education, transportation, communication, recreation, institutionalization, health services, voting, and *access to public services.*" This finding, together with the extensive record of disability discrimination that underlies it, makes clear beyond peradventure [doubt] that inadequate provision of public services and access to public facilities was an appropriate subject for prophylactic legislation.

Response to Unequal Treatment

The only question that remains is whether Title II is an appropriate response to this history and pattern of unequal treatment. At the outset, we must determine the scope of that inquiry. Title II—unlike RFRA [Religious Freedom Restoration Act], the Patent Remedy Act, and the other statutes we have reviewed for validity under §5—reaches a wide array of official conduct in an effort to enforce an equally wide array of constitutional guarantees. Petitioner urges us both to examine the broad range of Title II's applications all at once, and to treat that breadth as a mark of the law's invalidity. According to petitioner, the fact that Title II applies not only to public education and voting-booth access but also to seating at state-owned hockey rinks indicates that Title II is not appropriately tailored to serve its objectives. But nothing in our case law requires us to consider Title II, with its wide variety of applications, as an undifferentiated whole. Whatever might be said about Title II's other applications, the question presented in this case is not whether Congress can validly subject the States to private suits for money damages for failing to provide reasonable access to hockey rinks, or even to voting booths, but whether Congress had the power under §5 to enforce the constitutional right of access to the courts. Because we find that Title II unquestionably is valid §5 legislation as it applies to the class of cases implicating the accessibility of judicial services, we need go no further.

Congress' chosen remedy for the pattern of exclusion and discrimination described above, Title II's requirement of program accessibility, is congruent and proportional to its object of enforcing the right of access to the courts. The unequal treatment of disabled persons in the administration of judicial services has a long history, and has persisted despite several legislative efforts to remedy the problem of disability discrimination. Faced with considerable evidence of the shortcomings of previous legislative responses, Congress was justified in concluding that this "difficult and intractable proble[m]" warranted "added prophylactic measures in response."

The remedy Congress chose is nevertheless a limited one. Recognizing that failure to accommodate persons with disabilities will often have the same practical effect as outright exclusion, Congress required the States to take reasonable measures to remove architectural and other barriers to accessibility. But Title II does not require States to employ any and all means to make judicial services accessible to persons with disabilities, and it does not require States to compromise their essential eligibility criteria for public programs. It requires only "reasonable modifications" that would not fundamentally alter the nature of the service provided, and only when the individual seeking modification is otherwise eligible for the service. As Title II's implementing regulations make clear, the reasonable modification requirement can be satisfied in a number of ways. In the case of facilities built or altered after 1992, the regulations require compliance with specific architectural accessibility standards. But in the case of older facilities, for which structural change is likely to be more difficult, a public entity may comply with Title II by adopting a variety of less costly measures, including relocating services to alternative, accessible sites and assigning aides to assist persons with disabilities in accessing services. Only if these measures are ineffective in achieving accessibility is the public entity required to make reasonable structural changes. And in no event is the entity required to undertake measures that would impose an undue financial or administrative burden, threaten historic preservation interests, or effect a fundamental alteration in the nature of the service.

This duty to accommodate is perfectly consistent with the well-established due process principle that, "within the limits of practicability, a State must afford to all individuals a meaningful opportunity to be heard" in its courts. Our cases have recognized a number of affirmative obligations that flow from this principle: the duty to waive filing fees in certain family-law and criminal cases, the duty to provide transcripts to criminal defendants seeking review of their convictions, and the duty to provide counsel to certain criminal defendants. Each of these cases makes clear that ordinary considerations of cost and convenience alone cannot justify a State's failure to provide individuals with a meaningful right of access to the courts. Judged against this backdrop, Title II's affirmative obligation to accommodate persons with disabilities in the administration of justice cannot be said to be "so out of proportion to a supposed remedial or preventive object that it cannot be understood as responsive to, or designed to prevent, unconstitutional behavior." It is, rather, a reasonable prophylactic measure, reasonably targeted to a legitimate end.

For these reasons, we conclude that Title II, as it applies to the class of cases implicating the fundamental right of access to the courts, constitutes a valid exercise of Congress' §5 authority to enforce the guarantees of the Fourteenth Amendment. The judgment of the Court of Appeals is therefore affirmed.

"We have never held that a person has a constitutional *right to make his way into a courtroom without any external assistance.*"

Dissenting Opinion: The Majority Ruling Is Inconsistent with Prior Decisions

William Rehnquist

William Rehnquist was nominated to the Supreme Court in 1971 by President Richard Nixon. After serving as an associate justice for fifteen years, he was nominated in 1986 by President Ronald Reagan to be chief justice of the United States. In his dissent in the case of Tennessee v. Lane and Jones, *he rejects the majority opinion that when it comes to the courts, states must follow Title II of the Americans with Disabilities Act, which guarantees accessibility of public facilities and services, or be subject to lawsuits from individuals. Rehnquist argues that the majority's opinion was inconsistent with the result the Court reached in* Alabama v. Garrett (2001), *in which it ruled that Congress had acted unconstitutionally in allowing citizens to sue states for disability discrimination under the Fourteenth Amendment's Equal Protection Clause. Rehnquist also objects to the majority's decision to limit the legal inquiry to the applicability of the law to courthouses alone because in his view the law applies to all services, programs, or activities of any public entity. Even if this narrowed focus is granted, he says, there was not*

William Rehnquist, dissenting opinion, *Tennessee v. Lane and Jones*, U.S. Supreme Court, 2004.

enough evidence to suggest that Congress viewed Title II as a means of remedying violations of due process. Further, he insists that there is no evidence to suggest that people with disabilities have been discriminated against in the courts or denied their constitutional rights, since they have not been denied the opportunity to be heard in civil cases, unconstitutionally excluded from jury service, or denied the right to attend criminal trials. The Court, he says, has never held that there is a constitutional right to make one's way into a courtroom without assistance, therefore inaccessible courthouses do not in themselves create constitutional violations.

In *Board of Trustees of Univ. of Ala. v. Garrett,* we held that Congress did not validly abrogate States' Eleventh Amendment immunity when it enacted Title I of the Americans with Disabilities Act of 1990 (ADA). Today, the Court concludes that Title II of that Act does validly abrogate that immunity, at least insofar "as it applies to the class of cases, implicating the fundamental right of access to the courts." Because today's decision is irreconcilable with *Garrett* and the well-established principles it embodies, I dissent. . . .

Evidence of Discrimination Is Irrelevant

Rather than limiting its discussion of constitutional violations to the due process rights on which it ultimately relies, the majority sets out on a wide-ranging account of societal discrimination against the disabled. This digression recounts historical discrimination against the disabled through institutionalization laws, restrictions on marriage, voting, and public education, conditions in mental hospitals, and various other forms of unequal treatment in the administration of public programs and services. Some of this evidence would be relevant if the Court were considering the constitutionality of the statute as a whole; but the Court rejects that approach in favor of a narrower "as-applied" inquiry. We discounted much the same type of outdated, generalized evidence in *Garrett* as unsupportive of Title I's ban on employment discrimination. The evidence here is likewise irrelevant to Title II's purported enforcement of Due Process access-to-the-courts rights.

Even if it were proper to consider this broader category of evidence, much of it does not concern *unconstitutional* action by the *States*. The bulk of the Court's evidence concerns discrimination by nonstate governments, rather than the States themselves. We have repeatedly held that such evidence is irrelevant to the inquiry whether Congress has validly abrogated Eleventh Amendment immunity, a privilege enjoyed only by the sovereign States. Moreover, the majority today cites the same congressional task force evidence we rejected in *Garrett*. As in *Garrett*, this "unexamined, anecdotal" evidence does not suffice. Most of the brief anecdotes do not involve States at all, and those that do are not sufficiently detailed to determine whether the instances of "unequal treatment" were irrational, and thus unconstitutional. Therefore, even outside the "access to the courts" context, the Court identifies few, if any, constitutional violations perpetrated by the States against disabled persons.

With respect to the due process "access to the courts" rights on which the Court ultimately relies, Congress' failure to identify a pattern of actual constitutional violations by the States is even more striking. Indeed, there is *nothing* in the legislative record or statutory findings to indicate that disabled persons were systematically denied the right to be present at criminal trials, denied the meaningful opportunity to be heard in civil cases, unconstitutionally excluded from jury service, or denied the right to attend criminal trials. . . .

Even if the anecdotal evidence and conclusory statements relied on by the majority could be properly considered, the mere existence of an architecturally "inaccessible" courthouse—*i.e.*, one a disabled person cannot utilize without assistance—does not state a constitutional violation. A violation of due process occurs only when a person is actually denied the constitutional right to access a given judicial proceeding. We have never held that a person has a *constitutional* right to make his way into a courtroom without any external assistance. Indeed, the fact that the State may need to assist an individual to attend a hearing has no bearing on whether the individual successfully exercises his due process right to be present at the proceeding. Nor does an "inaccessible" courthouse violate the Equal Protection Clause, unless it is irrational for the State not to alter the courthouse to make it "accessible." But financial considerations almost always furnish a rational basis for a State to decline to make those alterations. Thus, evidence regarding inaccessible courthouses, because it is not evidence of constitutional violations, provides no basis to abrogate States' sovereign immunity.

The near-total lack of actual constitutional violations in the congressional record is reminiscent of *Garrett,* wherein we found that the same type of minimal anecdotal evidence "f[e]ll far short of even suggesting the pattern of unconstitutional [state action] on which §5 legislation must be based."

The barren record here should likewise be fatal to the majority's holding that Title II is valid legislation enforcing due process rights that involve access to the courts. This conclusion gains even more support when Title II's nonexistent record of constitutional violations is compared with legislation that we have sustained as valid §5 enforcement legislation. Accordingly, Title II can only be understood as a congressional attempt to "rewrite the Fourteenth Amendment law laid down by this Court," rather than a legitimate effort to remedy or prevent state violations of that Amendment.

> "Lane ... has sent a signal to the dis-
> ability rights community that the ADA
> has not become a dead letter yet."

The *Lane* Ruling
Reinvigorated the ADA

Russell Powell

*Russell Powell is an associate professor of law at Seattle Univer-
sity School of Law. In the following essay, he reviews the state of
disability law under the Americans with Disabilities Act (ADA),
with particular attention to* Tennessee v. Lane and Jones. *In*
Lane, *the Court affirmed that Congress validly exercised its
power when it made states subject to suits under the ADA, at
least with regard to limitations on access to courts. The Court
upheld lower court findings that two mobility-impaired plaintiffs, George Lane and Beverly Jones were entitled to sue the state
of Tennessee for its failure to make accessible the upper floors in
state courthouses. Powell says that while the* Lane *decision addresses Title II of the ADA, which outlines restrictions on state
discrimination, it also has implications for the act as a whole.
The ruling reflects a shift in the way the court views the ADA
and disability cases, creating an opportunity for greater dialogue
about the goals of the ADA and justice for people with disabilities.*

When the Americans with Disabilities Act (the "Act" or
the "ADA") was enacted in 1990, many disability rights
advocates expected that it would usher in a new era of equal

Russell Powell, "Beyond *Lane*: Who Is Protected by the Americans with Disabilities Act,
Who Should Be?" *Denver University Law Review*, vol. 82, Fall 2004, pp. 25–26, 37–39, 56.
Reproduced by permission of the author.

opportunity and acceptance for people with disabilities. Written in the tradition of both the Rehabilitation Act of 1973 and the Civil Rights Act of 1964, the ADA reflected the ideal of distributive justice in its mandate to both counter discrimination and provide accommodation; however, the courts gradually narrowed its coverage. Some empirical studies assert that the ADA actually caused a decline in the rate of employment among people with disabilities. By early 2000, some scholars predicted that the ADA would fade into obscurity as an ill-conceived relic that failed to adequately anticipate social costs and the rational choices of employers and people with disabilities.

Broad Implications of *Lane*

However, the ADA received new vigor from the Supreme Court with the May 2004 opinion, *Tennessee v. Lane*. In a 5-4 decision, the Court affirmed that Congress validly exercised its power when it subjected states to suits under the ADA, at least with regard to limitations on access to courts. While the decision addresses Title II of the ADA, it does have broader implications for the Act as a whole. *Lane* reflects a significant shift in the ethical paradigm used by the Court to decide ADA cases and creates the opportunity to re-open dialogue about the real policy goals of the ADA and broader questions of justice for those with disabilities. Analysis of the measurable impact of the ADA continues and results in sometimes conflicting assertions. But whatever conclusions are ultimately proven, the question of our policy goals and our conception of justice for people with disabilities must be distinguished from the judicial and legislative tools intended to achieve those goals.

The ADA's legislative history makes it clear that it was intended to address the social issues associated with discrimination as well as accessibility issues for those with physical impairments. The Supreme Court's emphasis on impairment and the notion of a discrete and insular minority found in civil rights legislation has transformed the scope of the ADA found in its plain meaning. The result is that some claimants who fall within the intended and literal scope of the ADA do not receive the benefit of its protection. Furthermore, states have largely been exempted from the requirements of the ADA, *Lane* notwithstanding.

Under Title I (the ADA's employment provisions), even those who can make a successful claim may be caught in the catch-22 of winning a case but being terminated because their impairment makes them unemployable. Although those who care for the disabled are not expressly covered by any part of the ADA, it is arguable that they constitute a vulnerable class which should receive fair compensation and perhaps legal protections under the ADA (though admittedly this might be more appropriately addressed under a different legislative aegis). For these reasons, this paper recommends a reconsideration of the ADA's goals and a review of its effectiveness. While such a project is broader than the scope of this paper, its ultimate conclusions may necessitate changes in disability policy and justify substantial amendments to the ADA which would better-serve the original legislative intent and the interests of the disabled. . . .

Facts of the Case

[In *Tennessee v. Lane,*] the respondents, George Lane and Beverly Jones, are both paraplegics who use wheelchairs. Lane crawled up two flights of stairs to make an appearance to respond to criminal charges in a court-house that had no elevator. When he returned for a hearing, he refused either to crawl or be carried to the courtroom and was arrested and jailed for failure to appear. Beverly Jones, a certified court reporter who relied on access to courtrooms for her livelihood and was unable to gain access to a number of county courthouses, joined in the action challenging the State of Tennessee pursuant to Title II of the ADA.

Tennessee moved to dismiss the suit at the District Court level on the grounds of Eleventh Amendment immunity. The District Court denied the motion, and Tennessee appealed the decision to the Sixth Circuit Court of Appeals. The Sixth Circuit ultimately affirmed the denial of dismissal on due process grounds. Since the Supreme Court had ruled in *Bd. of Tr. of the Univ. of Ala. v. Garrett* that states were immune from Title I liability despite equal protection concerns, some commentators expected Eleventh Amendment immunity to be extended to all Title II suits. However, in a 5-4 decision drafted by Justice [John Paul] Stevens, the Supreme Court ruled that the fundamental right to court access is a valid justification for Congress' enactment of Title II pursuant to its authority under section 5 of the Fourteenth Amendment.

The Court applied the two-part test adopted in *Kimel v. Florida Bd. of Regents* that requires Congress to unequivocally express its intent to abrogate [abolish] state immunity and act pursuant to valid constitutional authority in rejecting the Eleventh Amendment challenge. Title II itself constituted unequivocal intent to abrogate immunity, but the question of valid authority implicated the test in *City of Boerne v. Flores*, which sets out the standard for permissible remedial legislation in these cases. The rule allows remedial legislation so long as it is "congruen[t] and proportional[]" to the threatened injury. Given the history and pattern of discrimination against the disabled and the compelling interest in a fundamental due process right, the Supreme Court upheld Title II with regard to states at least in cases involving access to courts. It is not clear whether Title II is enforceable against states in other settings.

A Reaction to Indignity

Although *Lane* is primarily an Eleventh Amendment case, it does have broader implications for other categories of ADA litigation. It has sent a signal to the disability rights community that the ADA has not become a dead letter yet. The majority in *Lane* includes those Justices who are typically considered the more liberal members of the Court (Justices Stevens, [David] Souter, [Ruth Bader] Ginsburg and [Stephen] Breyer), along with Justice [Sandra Day] O'Connor, and seems to represent a shift away from the trend toward narrowing the scope of the ADA, at least with respect to the due process right to court access. However, it is not clear whether this rule will apply to Title II suits under any other circumstances. Such a specific carve-out may not contribute to greater predictability and efficiency in ADA litigation, but it does represent a response to facts that demonstrated an extreme case of the sorts of indignity people with disabilities have been subjected to in this country—with limited or no legal recourse. As the clear deciding vote, Justice O'Connor's position is almost certainly a reaction to this extreme sort of indignity. While not a formalist in the sense of more conservative members of the Court, among her colleagues, Justice O'Connor is among the most consistent supporters of states' rights. Thus, her decision to abrogate Eleventh Amendment immunity in this case indicates a competing, more important value.

Justices [Clarence] Thomas and [Anthony] Kennedy join Chief Justice [William] Rehnquist in his dissent. In it they dispute the majority's conclusions in applying the *Boerne* test as reaffirmed in *Garrett*. On the sole basis of formalism, the argument is likely more consistent with Eleventh Amendment jurisprudence than the majority position. Justice [Antonin] Scalia's dissent objects to the "congruence and proportionality test" generally as a "flabby" test. His concerns are characteristically both pragmatic and textual. . . .

ADA Needs Amendment

Our comprehensive approach to disability must distinguish between cases that address functional issues of access based on impairment and discrimination issues based on stigma. This would return us to the social model apparently intended by Congress, at least with regard to discrimination cases. . . .

New legislation must be clearly drafted to unequivocally and strategically define the categories of those who should be protected under the ADA as well as demonstrate a clear history of discrimination against the disabled. Legislation must aggressively address the challenges to Congressional authority posed by recent Supreme Court cases within the framework of those decisions in the context of federalism.

The ADA was intended to promote justice for the disabled. It has become a model for many nations. Unfortunately, the reach of the ADA has been gradually eroded by court decisions. Perhaps without even intending it, the Supreme Court has created a legal framework that is filled with contradictions and denies justice to the intended beneficiaries of the legislation. If the ADA is not amended, its effectiveness as an antidiscrimination law will likely continue to diminish, even if cases such as *Lane* occasionally enforce its provisions in narrow circumstances.

"The four dissenters in Lane got the
main question right."

The Court Was Mistaken
in Its *Lane* Ruling

Robert A. Levy

Robert A. Levy is chairman of the Cato Institute's board of directors. In the following essay, he says that Tennessee v. Lane
and Jones, *in which the Court decided that two mobility-impaired plaintiffs could sue the state for failure to make courthouses accessible to people with disabilities, was a case about sovereign immunity and congressional power. He says that the Court was correct on the immunity question, but for the wrong reason. Tennessee, he says, should not have been entitled to immunity, but not because its claim was revoked by Congress but rather because the Eleventh Amendment does not confer immunity in federal question cases. On the congressional power question, says Levy, the Court mistakenly found legislative authority under section five of the Fourteenth Amendment to enact Title II of the Americans with Disabilities Act. Levy contends that given the facts in Lane, that power does not exist. He shows where the dissenters were correct in their assessment that there is no constitutional power to compel states to provide access by disabled persons to all of the "services, programs, or activities of a public entity."*

The underlying statute at issue in [*Tennessee v. Lane and Jones*] was the Americans with Disabilities Act of 1990

Robert A. Levy, "*Tennessee v. Lane*: How Illegitimate Power Negated Non-Existent Immunity," *Cato Supreme Court Review*, 2004, pp. 162–3, 168–78. Republished with permission of Cato Institute, conveyed through Copyright Clearance Center, Inc.

(ADA), which states in Title II that "no qualified individual with a disability shall, by reason of such disability, be excluded from participation in or denied the benefits of the services, programs or activities of a public entity." Plaintiffs Beverly Jones and George Lane, both paraplegics, sued the state of Tennessee, contending that they were refused access to, and the services of, the state court system on account of their disability. Jones is a court reporter who asserted that she lost work because some county court-houses are not wheelchair-accessible. Lane alleged more agonizing facts. He was charged with a criminal traffic offense and had to crawl up two flights of stairs to reach the courtroom. At a subsequent hearing, he declined a second opportunity to crawl or be carried, and then rejected an offer to move all proceedings to a handicapped-accessible courtroom in a nearby town. As a result, Lane was arrested and jailed for failing to appear at his hearing.

The trial court denied Tennessee's motion to dismiss claims by Jones and Lane on immunity grounds. Tennessee then asked the U.S. Court of Appeals for the Sixth Circuit to reverse. At first, the Sixth Circuit delayed review until the Supreme Court could rule in a then-pending Eleventh Amendment case, *Board of Trustees of the University of Alabama v. Garrett*, which also involved the ADA (albeit Title I, prohibiting employment discrimination against the disabled.) But then the Sixth Circuit changed its mind: The court of appeals decided that *Garrett* did not control the outcome in *Lane* after all. That's because *Garrett* was an equal protection case alleging employment discrimination against a particular class—the disabled—in violation of the ADA's Title I. *Lane*, by contrast, was a Title II case based on denial of courtroom access, which was deemed to be a due process issue. Based in part on that distinction, the Sixth Circuit upheld the trial court's refusal to dismiss *Lane*.

Supreme Court's Findings

The Supreme Court agreed with the Sixth Circuit. Essentially, the Supreme Court adopted this logic:

- Under the Eleventh Amendment, Tennessee is entitled to sovereign immunity against suits for money damages.

- Congress can abrogate Tennessee's sovereign immunity if, among other things, it clearly expresses an intent to do so. The Court found that Congress had unambiguously declared its intent in the ADA.

- However, Congress also must base its abrogation of immunity on some constitutional authority. When it passed the ADA, Congress cited both the Commerce Clause and the Fourteenth Amendment as its source of authority. But an earlier Supreme Court case held that Congress, when it enacts legislation under the Commerce Clause, cannot abrogate [abolish] Eleventh Amendment immunity. The Court, therefore, turned to section 5 of the Fourteenth Amendment.

- The Court held Congress *can* abrogate immunity when it enacts legislation to enforce the Fourteenth Amendment's Due Process and Equal Protection Clauses, provided that the means adopted are "congruent and proportional" to the underlying harm. In *Lane*, said the Court, those conditions were met by Title II of the ADA.

The Case Against Sovereign Immunity

Beginning in 1890 and concluding with an unbroken string of seven cases from 1996 through 2002, the Supreme Court enlarged the doctrine of sovereign immunity, which bars most private lawsuits against non-consenting state governments for money damages. Along the way, the Court ignored the plain text of the Eleventh Amendment: "The Judicial power of the United States shall not be construed to extend to any suit in law or equity, commenced or prosecuted against one of the United States by Citizens of another State, or by Citizens or Subjects of any Foreign State." . . .

The Court has acknowledged only one new exemption from its ballooning immunity doctrine: States remain vulnerable to private suits pursuant to federal laws that enforce the Fourteenth Amendment. But then, in four cases from 1999 through 2001, the Court steadily chipped away at that exemption. . . .

[T]he Court's ever-widening immunity doctrine was broadened to bar suits by private parties against a state in a federal administrative agency. The conservative majority in that case, *Federal Maritime Commission v. South Carolina State Ports Authority*, asserted that the "central purpose" of sovereign immunity "is to accord the States the respect owed them as joint sovereigns." In other words, the primary reason for immunity is to give the states the dignity that their sovereign status entails.

But if state dignity is the justification for sovereign immunity, what can explain the numerous exceptions that have been carved out? A state can be sued by the federal government or another state. Political subdivisions, school boards, and municipalities, which are creations of the state, can be sued under the Eleventh Amendment. So can state officials in their personal capacity. And both [*Nevada Department of Human Resources v. Hibbs et al.*] (2003) and *Lane* (2004) now confirm that a state can be sued by private individuals in certain enforcement actions under the Fourteenth Amendment.

The relevant legislation in *Hibbs* was the Family Medical Leave Act (FMLA), which grants unpaid leave when an employee's parent, child, or spouse is seriously ill. The FMLA was designed to address lingering gender discrimination in the workplace. Congress found that women were disproportionately burdened by having to take care of sick family members. Because the alleged discrimination was based on gender, which the Court gives heightened review, not the minimal scrutiny applied to age- or disability-based discrimination, "it was easier for Congress to show a pattern of state constitutional violations."

Like *Hibbs*, *Lane* was a case in which the Court had an easier time finding state misconduct that rose to the level of a constitutional infraction. In *Lane*, however, the Court's heightened scrutiny was not attributable to discrimination on the basis of a suspect class. Instead, the Court's rationale was based on due process, and the increased scrutiny derived from alleged denial of a "fundamental" right—access to the court.

The Trouble with Sovereign Immunity

By abrogating Tennessee's sovereign immunity, *Lane* produced the right result—even though for the wrong reason. Regrettably, the Court missed its ninth opportunity in eight years to affirm that compensating injured parties and deterring state misbehavior takes precedence over safeguarding government bank accounts. A free society cannot subordinate the rights of individuals to the "dignity" of state governments—not even with the noble aim of inhibiting federal power.

A proper understanding of the role of government dictates that the Eleventh Amendment be construed narrowly. Clearly, that is not what the Court had done pre-*Hibbs*. By its extra-textual reading of the amendment, the Court took the common law concept of sovereign immunity, dubious on its own terms, and constitutionalized it. Concern for state dignity superseded the rights of individuals, relegated by judicial edict to the bottom of the pecking order. Essentially, the [William] Rehnquist Court had embraced the appalling notion that states can violate individual rights without being held accountable for monetary losses associated with personal injuries.

In its defense, the Court proceeded with the best of intentions—to restrain a Congress that has flouted the doctrine of enumerated powers and established a pervasive regulatory and redistributive state that threatens individual liberty. The federal government has wormed its way into virtually every aspect of our lives—imposing rules to control a broad array of human endeavor, exacting tribute from anyone, for almost any purpose, then dispensing the proceeds to anyone else. No doubt, the Court's steps to curtail Congress's seemingly boundless powers were long overdue.

But, while the Rehnquist Court justifiably tried to slow down the federal juggernaut, it went about it in the wrong manner. The proper remedy is to attack unconstitutional statutes on their merits, not to pretend that federal law can't be invoked by individuals against state governments when damages are sought. . . .

The effect of sovereign immunity is to place the government above the law and to ensure that some individuals will be unable to obtain redress for injuries. That's simply not acceptable. In a free society, the "dignity" of state governments cannot be permitted to trump the rights of individual Americans.

Perhaps the Constitution would be a more liberating document if the Eleventh Amendment had never been ratified. But, of course, it was ratified in 1795, and the Court is stuck with it. That does not, however, obligate the Court to extend the reach of the amendment by reading more into it than can possibly be justified by its unambiguous text. . . .

In *Hibbs*, Justice [Anthony] Kennedy, joined in dissent by Justices [Antonin] Scalia and [Clarence] Thomas, questioned whether the states had "engaged in a pattern of unlawful conduct which warrants the remedy of opening state treasuries to private suits." He remarked on the Court's inability to adduce evidence of alleged discrimination and on "the inescapable fact that the federal scheme is not a remedy but a benefit program." Justice Scalia, in a separate dissent, warned against "guilt by association, enabling the sovereignty of one State to be abridged . . . because of violations by another State . . . or even by 49 other States."

The same three justices dissented in *Lane*, along with Chief Justice Rehnquist. . . .

Rehnquist's Dissent

Rehnquist, joined by Kennedy and Thomas, argued that Title II of the ADA is not a valid section 5 enforcement action. Instead, like Title I in *Garrett*, Title II substantively redefines the rights protected by the Fourteenth Amendment. In reaching that conclusion, Rehnquist goes through the three-step process spelled out in *Boerne*: first, identify the rights at issue; second, examine the evidence cited by Congress to establish a pattern of violations; and third, consider whether the remedies created by Title II are congruent and proportional to the documented violations.

With respect to the rights at issue, Rehnquist observed that Title II goes beyond the equal protection concerns of Title I, which protects the disabled against irrational discrimination. Title II also purports to safeguard rights—such as courtroom access—that fall under the Due Process Clause. Specifically, Rehnquist pinpointed four due process rights cited by the majority: "(1) the right of the criminal defendant to be present at all critical stages of the trial; (2) the right of litigants to have a meaningful opportunity to be heard in judicial proceedings; (3) the right of the criminal defendant to trial by a jury composed of a fair cross section of the community; and (4) the public right of access to criminal proceedings."

Next, Rehnquist asked whether Congress had found a history and pattern of violations. His answer: an unequivocal "no." Although Congress, when it enacted the ADA, offered a wide-ranging account of societal discrimination against the disabled, the bulk of the evidence—mostly unexamined and anecdotal—concerned non-state government acts, which had been deemed irrelevant in prior sovereign immunity cases like *Garrett* and *Kimel* [*v. Florida Board of Regents*]. Some of that evidence might be relevant, stated Rehnquist, if the Court were reviewing Title II as a whole. But the Court had rejected that approach, preferring a narrower "as-applied" inquiry that focused only on courtroom access.

Even if Title II is viewed narrowly, Rehnquist insisted, "the mere existence of an architecturally 'inaccessible' court-house ... does not state a constitutional violation. A violation of due process occurs only when a person is actually denied the constitutional right to access a given judicial proceeding. We have never held that a person has a *constitutional* right to make his way into a courtroom without any external assistance."

Finally, Rehnquist explored the congruence and proportionality of Title II's remedial provisions. In its findings, Congress had made it clear that Title II attacked discrimination in all areas of public services, as well as the "discriminatory effect" of "architectural, transportation, and communication barriers." Rehnquist maintained that those broad terms go beyond arguable constitutional violations. Title II is not tailored to protect *just* courtroom access. Instead, it covers all services, programs, and activities provided by a public entity. As Rehnquist noted, a "requirement of accommodation for the disabled at a state-owned amusement park or sports stadium ... bears no permissible prophylactic relationship to enabling disabled persons to exercise their fundamental constitutional rights."

Put somewhat differently, Rehnquist considered the coverage of Title II to be massively overbroad—a problem that the majority claimed to have cured with its "as-applied" approach, limited to courtroom access. Rehnquist would sooner have invalidated Title II on a "facial" basis because of its many un-

constitutional applications, even if he were to concede that
Title II's application to Lane's particular challenge might be
constitutional.

To be sure, the Court typically disfavors facial, or over-
breadth, challenges—preferring to avoid constitutional con-
frontations by contracting the reach of congressional statutes.
In this instance, however, Rehnquist argued persuasively that
the Court's as-applied test cannot be harmonized with *Boerne*'s
test for congruence and proportionality. After all, how can the
majority assert, on one hand, that Title II must be construed
narrowly because it would otherwise restrict state conduct
that is constitutionally permissible; then, on the other hand,
assert that the remedies provided by Title II are congruent
and proportional to documented violations of constitutional
rights?

The majority gets away with that legerdemain [sleight of
hand] by positing "a hypothetical statute, never enacted by
Congress, that applies only to courthouses. The effect is to rig
the congruence-and-proportionality test by artificially con-
stricting the scope of the statute to closely mirror a recognized
constitutional right." That bogus approach, said Rehnquist, becomes a test of whether the Court can visualize an imaginary
statute that is narrow enough to constitute valid prophylactic
legislation.

Scalia's Dissent

Justice Scalia agreed with the chief justice. He too believed
that the majority flouted the congruence and proportionality
standard. But he filed a separate dissent in *Lane* to push that
message further than the other dissenters were willing to go.
Despite joining the Court's opinion in *Boerne*, Scalia rejected
the congruence and proportionality test—not only because it
is incompatible with the Court's as-applied maneuver in *Lane*,
but also because he does not approve of "such malleable stan-

dards as 'proportionality,' because they have a way of turning into vehicles for the implementation of individual judges' policy preferences."

Scalia claimed to have yielded to the "lessons of experience. The 'congruence and proportionality' standard, like all such flabby tests, is a standing invitation to judicial arbitrariness and policy-driven decisionmaking. . . . Under it, the courts . . . must regularly check Congress's homework to make sure that it has identified sufficient constitutional violations to make its remedy congruent and proportional."

In its place, Scalia would substitute a different test, which appears in the text of section 5 of the Fourteenth Amendment. He would require Congress to "enforce" section 5, not to "go *beyond* the provisions of the Fourteenth Amendment to proscribe, prevent, or 'remedy' conduct that does not *itself* violate any provision of the Fourteenth Amendment." "So-called 'prophylactic legislation,'" states Scalia, "is reinforcement rather than enforcement."

Scalia conceded just two exceptions to his far-reaching proposal. First, he would authorize legislation that imposes rules directly related to the facilitation of enforcement—like reporting requirements, for example. Second, he would respect past decisions now well-settled in law and allow, on *stare decisis* [precedent] grounds, prophylactic measures to combat racial discrimination alone. That single practice, according to Scalia, was the issue in dispute when the Court expansively interpreted section 5. When congressional legislation was targeted at discrimination in other areas, the Court was more restrained.

Hereafter, advised Scalia, he will "leave it to Congress, under constraints no tighter than those of the Necessary and Proper Clause, to decide what measures are appropriate under § 5 to prevent or remedy racial discrimination by the States." But even in race cases, Scalia will insist that Congress can impose prophylactic legislation on those *particular* states, and no others, that have a history of relevant constitutional violations. In cases not directed at racial discrimination, Scalia will uphold only those statutes that enforce the provisions of the Fourteenth Amendment—that is, legislation that addresses actual or imminent constitutional violations, and does not proscribe state conduct that itself is constitutional, even to deter other conduct that may not be.

Although Rehnquist, Thomas, and Kennedy did not subscribe to Scalia's recommended overhaul of section 5 jurisprudence, the four dissenters in *Lane* got the main question right. There is no constitutional power under section 5 of the Fourteenth Amendment to compel states to provide access by disabled persons to all of the "services, programs or activities of a public entity." That's what Title II is about, and to interpret it narrowly—as if it meant access only to courtrooms—is to ignore its text and eviscerate the mandate in *Boerne* that section 5 legislation must be congruent and proportional to asserted injuries.

Organizations to Contact

The editors have compiled the following list of organizations concerned with the issues debated in this book. The descriptions are derived from materials provided by the organizations. All have publications or information available for interested readers. The list was compiled on the date of publication of the present volume; the information provided here may change. Be aware that many organizations take several weeks or longer to respond to inquiries, so allow as much time as possible.

**The American Association of People
with Disabilities (AAPD)**
1629 K Street NW, Suite 950, Washington, DC   20006
(202) 457-0046 • fax: (202) 457-0473
Web site: www.aapd.com

The American Association of People with Disabilities organizes the disability community to be a force for change—politically, socially, and economically—and recognizes the value of working in broad coalitions to foster unity, leadership, and impact. The organization's mission is to ensure economic and political empowerment of all people with disabilities; further the productivity, independence, full citizenship, and total integration of people with disabilities into all aspects of society; foster leadership among people with disabilities; support the full implementation and enforcement of disability nondiscrimination laws, particularly the Americans with Disabilities Act of 1990 and the Rehabilitation Act of 1973; provide information to the disability community; and educate the public and government policy makers regarding issues affecting people with disabilities.

The Arc
1010 Wayne Ave., Suite 650, Silver Spring, MD   20910
(301) 565-3842 • fax: (301) 565-3843

Web site: www.thearc.org

The Arc is the world's largest community-based organization of and for people with intellectual and developmental disabilities. It provides an array of services and support for families and individuals and includes over 140,000 members affiliated through more than 850 state and local chapters across the nation. The Arc is devoted to promoting and improving supports and services for all people with intellectual and developmental disabilities. The organization has many publications, including fact sheets and a family resource guide.

Bazelon Center for Mental Health Law
1101 Fifteenth Street NW, Suite 1212, Washington, DC   20005
(202) 467-5730 • fax: (202) 223-0409
Web site: www.bazelon.org

The mission of the Bazelon Center for Mental Health Law is to protect and advance the rights of adults and children who have mental disabilities. The organization's advocacy is based on the principle that every individual is entitled to choice and dignity. The Bazelon Center uses a coordinated approach of litigation, policy analysis, coalition building, public information, and technical support for local disability advocates. The center produces a variety of publications related to disability rights.

Cato Institute
1000 Massachusetts Ave. NW, Washington, DC   20001
(202) 842-0200 • fax: (202) 842-3490
Web site: www.cato.org

The Cato Institute is a nonpartisan public policy research foundation dedicated to promoting limited government and individual liberty. The institute believes the Americans with Disabilities Act is not effective and imposes unreasonable costs on businesses. The institute publishes the *Cato Journal, Cato's Letter* newsletter, the *Cato's Letter* essays, and numerous position papers, including "Handicapping Freedom: The Americans with Disabilities Act" and "The Unintended Consequences of the Americans with Disabilities Act."

Disability Rights Advocates (DRA)
2001 Center Street, 4th Floor, Berkeley, CA   94704-1204
(510) 665-8644 • fax: (510) 665-8511
Web site: www.dralegal.org

Disability Rights Advocates (DRA) is a nonprofit legal center whose mission is to ensure dignity, equality, and opportunity for people with all types of disabilities throughout the United States and worldwide. DRA's national advocacy work includes high-impact class action litigation on behalf of people with all types of disabilities, including mobility, hearing, vision, learning, and psychological. Through negotiation and litigation, DRA has made thousands of facilities throughout the country accessible and has enforced access rights for millions of people with disabilities in many key areas of life, including access to technology, education, employment, transportation, and health care. DRA also engages in nonlitigation advocacy throughout the country, including research and education projects focused on opening up access to schools, professions, and health care. DRA publishes a periodic statistical report, *Disability Watch*, that analyzes barriers and emerging issues facing people with disabilities. DRA also publishes various "Know Your Rights" handbooks designed to educate and assist people with disabilities in knowing and enforcing their civil rights.

Disability Rights Education and Defense Fund (DREDF)
2212 Sixth Street, Berkeley, CA   94710
(510) 644-2555 • fax: (510) 841-8645
e-mail: info@dredf.org
Web site: www.dredf.org

The Disability Rights Education and Defense Fund (DREDF), founded in 1979, is a leading national civil rights law and policy center directed by individuals with disabilities and parents who have children with disabilities. The mission of the DREDF is to advance the civil and human rights of people with disabilities through legal advocacy, training, education, and public policy and legislative development. The fund publishes reports, articles, pamphlets, and other materials, some of which are available on its Web site.

Easter Seals

233 S. Wacker Drive, Suite 2400, Chicago, IL   60606
(312) 726-6200 • fax: (312) 726-1494
Web site: www.easterseals.com

Easter Seals provides services, education, outreach, and advocacy to people living with autism and other disabilities. The groups offer medical rehabilitation services, employment training, and child care. Easter Seals has more than five hundred centers nationwide. Its Web site offers a legislative advocacy section and "facts about" section as well as firsthand accounts of people living with disabilities.

Families and Advocates Partnership for Education (FAPE)

8161 Normandale Blvd., Minneapolis, MN   55437-1044
(952) 838-9000 • fax: (952) 838-0199
e-mail: fape@fape.org
Web site: www.fape.org

Families and Advocates Partnership for Education is a partnership that aims to improve the educational outcomes for children with disabilities. It links families, advocates, and self-advocates to information about the Individuals with Disabilities Education Act (IDEA). The project is designed to address the information needs of the 6 million families in the United States whose children with disabilities receive special education services.

The National Coalition for Disability Rights (NCDR)

601 Pennsylvania Ave. NW, Suite 900S
Washington, DC   20004
(202) 448-9928
e-mail: jimward@ncdr.org
Web site: www.adawatch.org

The National Coalition for Disability Rights (NCDR) is a Washington, D.C.–based alliance of national, state, and local nonprofit organizations united to advance inclusion, social justice, and economic opportunity for children and adults with physical and mental disabilities. NCDR pools expertise, resources, and influence to build the capacity of nonprofit disability, civil rights, and social justice organizations to further its National Agenda for Disability Rights. With a particular emphasis on community organizing, preservation of disability social history, media and public outreach, NCDR promotes an understanding—impacting both social consciousness and public policy—of disability rights as essential civil and human rights.

Reason Foundation
3415 S. Sepulveda Blvd., Suite 400, Los Angeles, CA   90034
(310) 391-2245 • fax: (310) 391-4395
Web site: www.reason.org

The Reason Foundation is a national public policy research organization that promotes individual freedoms and libertarian principles. It believes that the Americans with Disabilities Act is too expensive to enforce. It publishes numerous publications, including the monthly *Privatization Watch* and the magazine *Reason*.

For Further Research

Books

Sharon N. Barnartt and Richard K. Scotch, *Disability Protests: Contentious Politics, 1970–1999*. Washington, DC: Gallaudet University Press, 2001.

H-Dirksen L. Bauman, *Open Your Eyes: Deaf Studies Talking*. Minneapolis: University of Minnesota Press, 2008.

Edwin Black, *War Against the Weak: Eugenics and America's Campaign to Create a Master Race*. Morrisville, NC: Dialog Press, 2008.

James I. Charlton, *Nothing About Us Without Us: Disability Oppression and Empowerment*. Berkeley and Los Angeles: University of California Press, 2000.

Luke J. Clements and Janet Read, *Disabled People and the Right to Life: The Protection and Violation of Disabled People's Most Basic Human Right*. New York: Routledge, 2008.

Diane Driedger, *The Last Civil Rights Movement*. New York: St. Martin's, 1989.

Doris Zames Fleischer and Frieda Zames, *The Disability Rights Movement: From Charity to Confrontation*. Philadelphia: Temple University Press, 2001.

L.O. Gostin and H.A. Beyer, eds., *Implementing the Americans with Disabilities Act: Rights and Responsibilities of All Americans*. Baltimore: Paul H. Brookes, 1993.

Robert M. Levy and Leonard S. Rubenstein, *The Rights of People with Mental Disabilities: The Authoritative ACLU Guide to the Rights of People with Mental Illness and Mental Retardation*. Carbondale: Southern Illinois University Press, 1996.

Paul K. Longmore, *Why I Burned My Book, and Other Essays on Disability*. Philadelphia: Temple University Press, 2003.

Paul K. Longmore and Lauri Umansky, eds., *The New Disability History: American Perspectives*. New York: New York University Press, 2001.

Richard K. Scotch, *From Good Will to Civil Rights: Transforming Federal Disability Policy*. 2nd ed. Philadelphia: Temple University Press, 2001.

Joseph P. Shapiro, *No Pity: People with Disabilities Forging a New Civil Rights Movement*. New York: Times Books, 1993.

Robert C. Smith, *A Case About Amy*. Philadelphia: Temple University Press, 1996.

James W. Trent Jr., *Inventing the Feeble Mind: A History of Mental Retardation in the United States*. Berkeley: University of California Press, 1994.

Periodicals

General

Garland E. Allen, "The Eugenics Record Office at Cold Spring Harbor, 1910–1940: An Essay in Institutional History," *Osiris*, 2nd ser., vol. 2, 1986.

Lyn Beekman, "Equal Education Through IDEA: How the Disabilities Education Act Works," *Family Advocate*, Winter 2009.

Robert D. Dinerstein, "'Every Picture Tells a Story, Don't It?' (1): The Complex Role of Narratives in Disability Cases," *Narrative*, January 2007.

David M. Engel and Frank W. Munger, "Narrative, Disability, and Identity," *Narrative*, January 2007.

Dahlia Lithwick, "What Are the Legal Rights of the Retarded?" *Slate*, July 12, 2001. www.slate.com.

Daniel H. Melvin II, "The Desegregation of Children with Disabilities," *DePaul Law Review*, Winter 1995.

Howard Moses, "The Americans with Disabilities Act of 1990," *American Rehabilitation*, Summer 1990.

Katherine Shaw, "The Disability Rights Movement—the ADA Today," *Momentum*, Fall 2008.

Pamela Wheaton Shorr, "Special Ed's Greatest Challenges . . . and Solutions: Here Are the Top Five Special Ed Issues That Affect School Administrators, with Resolutions for Each," *District Administration*, May 2006.

Buck v. Bell (1927)

J.H. Bell, "Eugenics of the Development of the Human Race," *Virginia Medical Monthly*, February 1931.

B. Branigin, "Warner Apologizes to Victims of Eugenics/ Woman Who Challenged Sterilizations Honored," *Washington Post*, May 3, 2002.

Paul A. Lombardo, "Carrie Buck's Pedigree," *Journal of Laboratory and Clinical Medicine*, vol. 138, 2001.

———, "Involuntary Sterilization in Virginia: From *Buck v. Bell* to *Poe v. Lynchburg*," *Developments in Mental Health Law*, July–September 1983.

———, "Taking Eugenics Seriously: Three Generations of ??? Are Enough?" *Florida State University Law Review*, Winter 2003.

———, "Three Generations, No Imbeciles: New Light on *Buck v. Bell*," *New York University Law Review*, vol. 60, no. 1, 1985.

Hendrick Hudson Central School District v. Rowley (1982)

Kenneth G. Anderson, "The Meaning of Appropriate Education to Handicapped Children Under the ECHA: The Impact of Rowley," *Southwestern University Law Review*, vol. 14, 1984.

Shelley A. Kroll, "Defining an Appropriate Education for Handicapped Children: *Board of Education v. Rowley*," *Syracuse Law Review*, vol. 34, 1983.

Barbara D. McGarry, "The *Rowley* Decision: How the Supreme Court Views the Education of Handicapped Children," *Journal of Visual Impairment & Blindness*, vol. 76, 1982.

Karen Meador, "What's Left After *Rowley*?: The Future of Advocacy in Special Education," *Exceptional Parent*, February 1983.

Bonnie P. Tucker, "*Board of Education of the Hendrick Hudson Central School District v. Rowley*: Utter Chaos," *Journal of Law and Education*, vol. 12, 1983.

Olmstead v. L.C. and E.W. (1999)

Samantha A. Dipolito, "*Olmstead v. L.C.*—Deinstitutionalization and Community Integration: An Awakening of the Nation's Conscience?" *Mercer Law Review*, Summer 2007.

Elizabeth Palley and Philip A. Rozario, "The Application of the *Olmstead* Decision on Housing and Eldercare," *Journal of Gerontological Social Work*, March–April 2007.

Michael L. Perlin, "'Their Promises of Paradise': Will *Olmstead v. L.C.* Resuscitate the Constitutional 'Least Restrictive Alternative' Principle in Mental Disability Law?" *Houston Law Review*, October 2000.

Dana E. Prescott, "Consent Decrees, the Enlightenment, and the 'Modern' Social Contract: A Case Study from *Bates, Olmstead*, and Maine's Separation of Powers Doctrine," *Maine Law Review*, April 2007.

Joel Teitelbaum, Taylor Burke, and Sara Rosenbaum, *"Olmstead v. L.C.* and the Americans with Disabilities Act: Implications for Public Health Policy and Practice," *Public Health Reports*, May–June 2004.

Tennessee v. Lane and Jones (2004)

Adam Cohen, "Can Disabled People Be Forced to Crawl Up the Courthouse Steps?" *New York Times*, January 11, 2004.

Mary Johnson, "Yes, but . . ." *Ragged Edge Online*, May 19, 2004. www.raggededgemagzine.com.

Dahlia Lithwick, "Crawling Up Stairs at a Courthouse Near You," *Slate*, January 13, 2004. www.slate.com.

Dave Reynolds, "Advocates Plan 'Stair Crawl' at Supreme Court," *Inclusion Daily Express*, January 8, 2004.

Warren Richey, "In Next Round, Will Disability Rights Be Broadened Further?" *Christian Science Monitor*, May 28, 2004.

Index

Polio epidemic, 15
Popenoe, Paul, 39
Powell, Russell, 172–177
Preadmission Screening and Resident Review (PASRR), 152
Prenatal screening, 55
Priddy, Albert, 21
Psychiatric hospitals, 17
Public buildings, accessibility requirements for, 18, 155, 163–165, 185–186
Public welfare, forced sterilization and, 26–27, 29–30

R

Reasonable-modifications regulation, 126–127, 143–144, 165–166
Rehabilitation Act (1973), 15–16
Rehnquist, William
  opinion of, in *Hendrick Hudson School District v. Rowley*, 16, 59, 61–73
  opinion of, in *Tennessee v. Lane and Jones*, 156, 168–171, 176, 184–186
Roosevelt, Eleanor, 17
Roosevelt, Franklin, 14
Roosevelt, Theodore, 14, 21
Rose v. Council for Better Education (1989), 92–93
Rosenberg, Linda, 150
Rowley, Amy June
  education of, 62–64, 81–82
  IEP of, 58, 63, 78–79, 107
  personal experiences of, 100–114
Rowley, Hendrick Hudson School District v. (1982). *See Hendrick Hudson School District v. Rowley* (1982)

S

Scalia, Antonin
  on *Nevada Department of Human Resources v. Hibbs et al.*, 183–184
  on *Tennessee v. Lane*, 186–188
School finance litigation, 91–92
Schools
  adequate yearly progress by, 95–96
  See also Education
Selective breeding, proponents of, 15
Sheie, Mary, 109
Shelton, R.G., 33
Siegel, Melvin, 151
Singer, Peter, 55
Sixth Amendment, 162–163
Skinner v. Oklahoma (1942), 22
Smith, R.C., 105, 109
Some educational benefit standard, 62, 68, 85–93, 96, 99
Sommers, Anne C., 53–56
South Carolina State Ports Authority, Federal Maritime Commission v. (2002), 181
Sovereign immunity
  case against, 180–182
  Eleventh Amendment and, 161–162, 169–171
  Fourteenth Amendment and, 187–188
  Tennessee v. Lane and, 155–157
  trouble with, 182–184
Special education
  definition of, 98
  standard for, set in *Rowley* case, 85–99

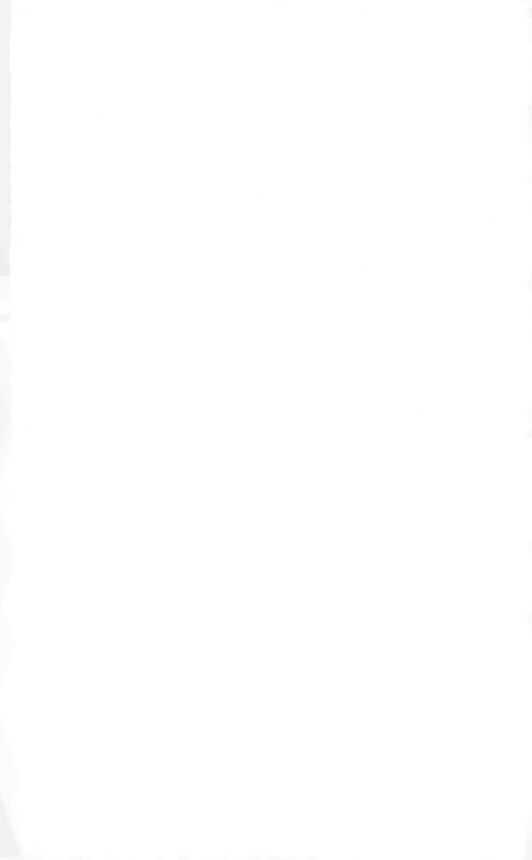